CHOCOLATE

Superfood of the Gods

Linda Woolven & Ted Snider

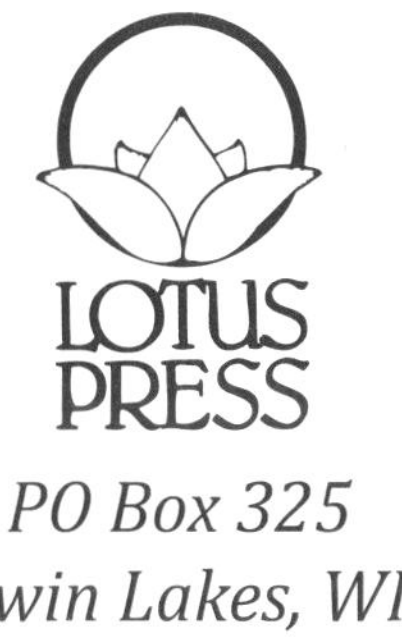

PO Box 325
Twin Lakes, WI

DISCLAIMER

This book is a reference work, not intended to diagnose, prescribe or treat. The information contained herein is in no way to be considered as a substitute for consulatation with a licensed health-care professional. It is designed to provide information on associated health, wellenss and dietary modalitites.

ISBN: 978-0-9406-7649-7
Library of Congress Number: 2018940521

Published by:

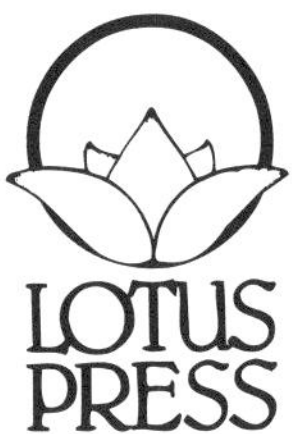

Lotus Press
P.O. Box 325
Twin Lakes, WI 53181 USA
800-824-6396 (toll free order phone)
262-889-8561 (office phone)
262-889-2461 (office fax)
www.lotuspress.com (website)
lotuspress@lotuspress.com (email)

Printed In USA

TABLE OF CONTENTS

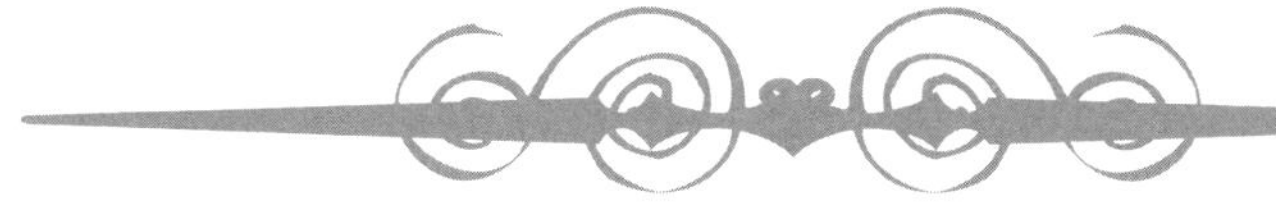

PART 7: CREATIVE COOKING WITH CHOCOLATE

Foreword

By Michael T. Murray, N.D.

Of all the foods available on planet Earth, perhaps the most magical (and fascinating) is chocolate. This delectably, seemingly addictive, food is packed full of unique compounds that exert a truly amazing constellation of effects within our body to promote health. Linda Woolven and Ted Snider have done an excellent job of detailing the magic of chocolate.

When I think of magic, I am reminded of something said by one of my all-time favorite authors, Sir Arthur Clarke. He is most famous for the novel *2001: A Space Odyssey*. Clarke made a statement that is quite relevant to the thought of chocolate and other foods being magical. He said, "Any sufficiently advanced technology is indistinguishable from magic." I can think of no more advanced technology than nature, and food is our direct link - a gift designed to nourish and heal us throughout our lifetime. And, there is no question that chocolate is one of nature's greatest gifts.

Though most enlightened individuals have a deep appreciation for the relationship between food and health, a new era of even greater acceptance of this undeniable link is emerging. It is an exciting time. As evident in this book, what is leading this paradigm shift to looking at food as the conduit to health as well as prescriptions to many diseases is increased scientific investigation. Science refers to the study of our environment and the greatest frontier of science is our relationship to food. It is quite an exciting time.

Would you believe me if I told you that scientists have discovered that your body has an internal medicine chest the size of a football field that is packed full of phenomenal and powerful remedies for inflammation, poor blood flow, high blood pressure, memory loss and virtually every other condition imaginable? Well, it is true, and it is chocolate's ability to impact this medicine chest that is what makes it such a powerful promoter of health.

This internal medicine chest is the lining of cells along the interior surface of all blood vessels. The technical term for this tissue is the endothelium and the cells that form this lining are called endothelial cells. From the heart to the smallest capillary, all vascular tissue has an endothelium. If all of the endothelial cells in the body were laid out flat, the endothelial surface area would be about the size of a football field. That is incredible to think about isn't it? Even more incredible is the way that chocolate and many other dietary factors can impact the endothelium. These effects are why chocolate has been referred to as nature's best medicine.

This book does an excellent job at reviewing these health benefits of chocolate in a truly inspiring manner. The takeaway message is that frequent consumption of chocolate or cacao, by impacting endothelial function, can go a very long way in helping to preserve vascular function, memory, and a positive mood as we age. Without question, in the right form, chocolate is a true super food. It is a perfect daily tonic for all ages, but especially baby boomers.

As you read this book, I urge you to open your imagination and be awed by what chocolate really does inspire in me – the awe and appreciation for the inherent magic of nature and the foods it creates. The more that I have learned about food and medicine, the greater my respect and appreciation for the harmony of nature has become.

This book is packed with series of observations, fascinating facts, and findings that can lead you on an amazing journey of discovery of the remarkable ways in which chocolate can impact your health. But, all of the information in the world means nothing if it does not lead to action. Through this book, my hope is that, by learning the wondrous ways in which chocolate promotes health, it will ignite or heighten your passion for focusing on foods that heal, instead of foods that harm, our health.

In good health,

Michael T. Murray, N.D.

Co-author, The Encyclopedia of Natural Medicine

DoctorMurray.com

PART 1:
Introduction

CHAPTER 1

A Brief History of Chocolate

It is not surprising that people love chocolate--it simply tastes so good--but what is surprising is how long people have been enjoying chocolate in its various forms and in how many different places it has been used. And just how good for you it is turning out to be.

Chocolate has been around for a very long time: some estimate 2000 years, some even longer. Sophie and Michael Coe say in their book, ***The True History of Chocolate***, that the earliest consumption of chocolate stretches back three or even four millennia to pre-Columbian cultures like the Olmec. By 1400 BCE, the sweet pulp of the cacao fruit, the part that surrounds the bean, had been fermented into an alcoholic beverage by the people living in Honduras, according to residue found on ancient pottery. Chocolate residues from as early as 1800 BCE have now been found in the Olmec capitol of San Lorenzo in Mexico. Evidence of the beginnings of chocolate's medicinal use goes all the way back to the Mesoamerican civilizations of the 7th century BCE.

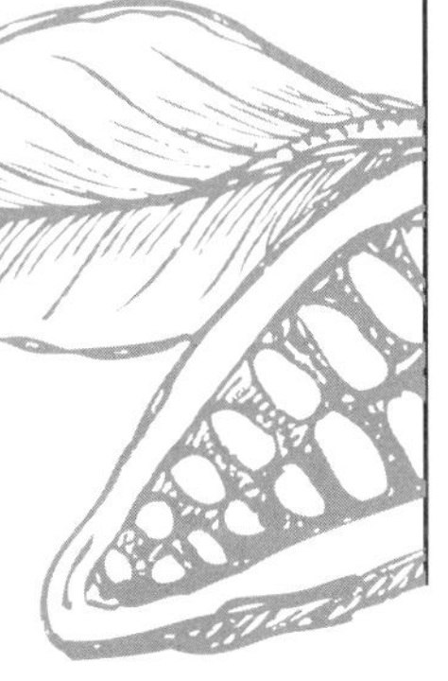

The word "chocolate" traces back to the ancient Aztecs, who drank a bitter brew made from cacao beans called ***xocoatl***. Cacao is the plant or its bean before it is processed into chocolate. Its Latin name, ***Theobroma cacao***, means food of the gods. Yet, it may have been discovered by accident. Researchers believe that chocolate was discovered when Central America Indians who were making beer from the pulp of the cacao seedpods found a new use for the byproduct.

Around 1100 BC, ancient beer makers were using seedpods of the cacao plant that were about the size of footballs to make their beer drinks. The pods were fermented and the seeds were discarded. The beer was, according to Rosemary Joyce, an anthropologist at University of California Berkley, a beer with a high kick. Three hundred years later, people began to use the discarded fermented seeds to make a non-alcoholic, very bitter and very prized beverage.

Although it seems to be hard to pin down exactly when chocolate was first made, it is very clear that from the time it was discovered, it was considered to be very valuable, even magical, and many thought it had divine powers. In pre-modern Latin America, cacao beans were considered valuable enough to use as currency. Both the Mayans and the Aztecs believed that the cacao bean was so important that it took on divine qualities and was used in sacred rituals surrounding birth, death and marriage. Legend even has it that Aztec sacrificial victims, who felt too sad before the ritual to join in the dancing, were given a gourd of chocolate (with the blood of the previous victims mixed in) to cheer them up. Now that must be some pretty powerful stuff to do that. Interestingly, even today, chocolate is often used to cheer people, especially women, up (without the blood or sacrifice!).

Chocolate was also used as trade for gems by the prehistoric Mesoamericans. Maybe that is because in prehistoric times, cacao, a tropical fruit that grows in Central and South America, was cultivated only in Mesoamerica, the region from Mexico to Costa Rica. Yet, it seems to have been traded from the 11th to the 14th centuries in New Mexico by the Mesoamericans and the Puebloans. Likely it was traded for turquoise. Trade also existed between the Mesoamericans and the Southwest peoples. Traces of chocolate were found at various sites in Pueblo Bonito in Chaco Canyon, New Mexico. And modern research has found traces of chocolate even among the farmers' vessels in this region. So even ordinary people had access to it. Chocolate was considered an important food on the menu at any special occasion by the Mesoamericans, much like the chocolate cakes, chocolate fountains, hot chocolate, boxes of chocolate and coffee mochas found for every occasion around the world today.

Why has chocolate always been so important? Well, it not only tastes great, but it is full of substances that benefit your health too. Chocolate contains ingredients that stimulate the heart and relax the airways, allowing people to breathe easier. It is also a good source of magnesium, which helps peoples' nerves, hearts, hormones, bones and mood. Mesoamericans gave chocolate to soldiers to pump them up before battle.

This incredibly delicious and important food did not make its way into Europe until Europe made its way into the Americas. And up until then, chocolate tended to be unsweetened.

So how did chocolate get discovered by the Europeans? According to legend, the Aztec king Montezuma welcomed the Spanish explorer Hernán Cortés with a banquet that included chocolate. He, unfortunately, mistook him for a reincarnated deity instead of the conquering invader he was. Cortés brought some cacao to King Charles of Spain in 1528. By the end of the sixteenth century, the first shipments of cacao were arriving in Spain.

But the bitterness of chocolate wasn't to the Europeans' taste. It was described in writings as "a bitter drink for pigs". So, it was mixed with honey or cane sugar, and it quickly became popular throughout Spain.

From then on, chocolate's popularity grew. By the 17th century, chocolate was believed to have nutritious, medicinal and even aphrodisiac properties (rumour has it that Casanova really liked chocolate and used it a lot), and it became a very fashionable drink for the wealthy throughout Europe. The invention of the steam engine made mass production possible by the late 1700s, and then chocolate was more readily available.

Its growing popularity made it a target for the Church. Because chocolate created euphoria, the Church declared that consuming chocolate invalidated religious fasts and that it could only be used for medicinal purposes.

By the eighteenth century, the famous botanist and physician Carl Linnaeus listed those medicinal uses still as nourishing and therapeutic and said it was effective for hypochondria, hemorrhoids and as an excellent aphrodisiac. Others called chocolate a universal medicine that stimulated warmth and the heart, got rid of gas, solved constipation, aided digestion, stimulated appetite, increased virility, slowed greying hair and prolonged life.

In the American Revolutionary war, it was included in the soldiers' rations and used as pay. And today, it is still huge business. In the United States alone, it is a more than four billion dollar industry. And the average person in the States eats half a pound or more of it per month.

All of this research into chocolate gives us new ideas as to what the ancients did with chocolate in the drinks and dishes they created and could even help give new ideas to today's chocolatiers and chefs.

Alice Medrich, author of ***Bittersweet: Recipes and Tales from a Life in Chocolate***, has said that "As a result, we get new ideas about using chocolate in savory as well as sweet dishes and about pairing the flavors of chocolate with other flavors, too. . . . New dishes and new trends are born. And new ideas spread from the most innovative and elite kitchens quickly, ultimately becoming products on supermarket shelves." And we'll do just that! After looking at all of the health research that has validated the ancient belief in chocolate's powerful health properties, we'll discover some new ideas and new dishes that explore chocolate, not only as a dessert treat, but as a featured ingredient in main courses.

CHAPTER 2

Flavonoids: The Story of Chocolate's Power

When you think of super foods, you usually think of foods that are green and taste like grass. But one of the most powerful super foods of all is dark and rich and delicious.

That chocolate is a healthy super food and not a junk food seemed inconceivable until the beginning of the 21st century, when the studies began, first, to trickle in and then, soon, to pour in to the medical journals.

We held off writing this book for many years, unable to believe that chocolate could be a health food. One of us has been a chocolate addict for years, and one of us became a convert while eating dark chocolate with chili and dark chocolate with ginger in Guatemala. It was a delicious food, but it belonged in books about desserts and not in books about health.

Perhaps the happiest day of my life was the day I read the first suggestion in ***The Journal of Nutrition*** that chocolate may increase antioxidant activity, improve cholesterol and reduce plaque formation and blood clotting: that it could be good for the heart. The early suggestion was cautious. The ***New York Times*** was excited enough to write a story on it in October of 2000, and the idea of chocolate as a health food entered the mainstream consciousness, but it cautioned that all the studies were preliminary. At that time, not a single double-blind, placebo-controlled

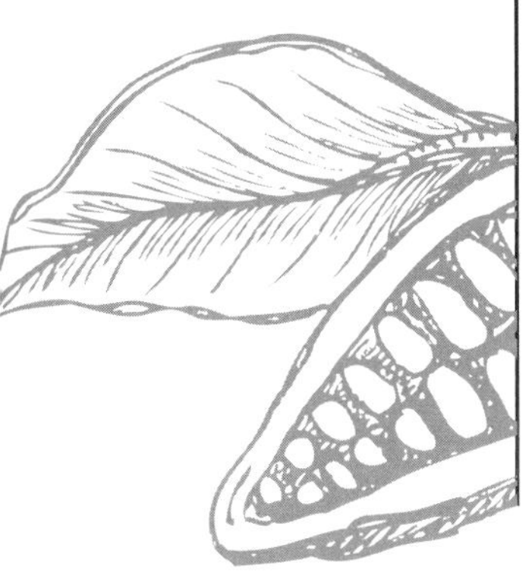

study had been done.

But all that has changed now. Our data base now contains hundreds of studies—many of them double-blind--on dark chocolate. The evidence is now so overwhelming that dark chocolate is an important health food that it is now crucial to put all that information together and put chocolate in its place as a food that you should be incorporating in your diet and not a food that you should be cutting back on.

You should be incorporating dark chocolate in your diet because it is loaded in flavonoids. Several famous foods are loaded in flavonoids, from blueberries to citrus fruit to red wine and green tea. But dark chocolate is a richer source of flavonoids than any of them.

Flavonoids make foods astringent and bitter. They are why red wine and green tea make your mouth feel dry; they are why the white of an orange is bitter. But chocolate is sweet not bitter. Well, the popular chocolate bars and chocolate candies are. Chocolate is not. As you sample the spectrum of chocolates from white chocolate to milk chocolate to increasingly dark chocolate and, finally, pure cocoa nibs, you'll notice the chocolate becoming more and more bitter. That's why many people prefer 70% dark chocolate bars to 85% dark chocolate bars, and why many people add sweetener to their hot chocolate. The Mayans and Aztecs, who were the first people to drink chocolate, called it ***xocoatl***, which means "bitter water." When you don't add milk and sugar, hot chocolate is bitter. The word "chocolate" comes from the word "***xocoatl***". So, our word "chocolate" means, not a sweet, but a bitter drink.

The more bitter the chocolate, the more flavonoids it contains. And the more flavonoids it contains, the better it is for you. So, white chocolate's not good for you at all. And dark chocolate is much better for you than milk chocolate.

The Many Colours of Chocolate

Chocolate begins as a large pod on a tree. Within each pod are an abundance of purple beans covered in a sweet, white pulp. The beans are purple because of the flavonoid content: the same reason why many antioxidant flavonoid rich foods, like blueberries, blackberries and dark grapes, are a dark purplish-blue. Those purple beans are then ground, roasted, shelled and fermented to make a chocolate liquor paste that is separated from the fat component of the beans, or nibs, that is known as cocoa butter. When you see a percentage on a chocolate bar, it is the cocoa liquor that is being measured. When you put cocoa butter back in with some sugar, you get dark chocolate. When you add milk, you get milk chocolate. So, the milk chocolate has less chocolate liquor in it and, so, less flavonoids. That is one of the reasons milk chocolate is less healthy. As you will see, there are others. White chocolate is just the cocoa butter with dairy and sweeteners but no cocoa liquor. So, white chocolate has no flavonoids at all and no health benefits.

When we talk about the health benefits of chocolate in this book, then, we are talking about dark chocolate: flavonoid rich dark chocolate. The substantial health benefits of dark chocolate are not derived from milk chocolate candy bars or white chocolate. The health benefits are also reduced if the chocolate you are eating has gone through a process called "dutching," which sometimes appears on the label as "processed with alkali." Dutching substantially reduces the level of the health providing flavonoids.

In addition to flavonoids, cocoa nibs contain significant amounts of the minerals magnesium, copper and iron. A 40g serving of 70% dark chocolate delivers about 10% of the recommended daily allowance of magnesium. Cocoa butter—the fat component of the cocoa bean—contains three kinds of fats: oleic acid (33%), palmitic acid (25%) and stearic acid (33%). But do not fear. Oleic acid is the same heart healthy fat found in olive oil. And palmitic acid and stearic acid, though they are saturated fats, do not act in your body like the saturated fats found in meat and dairy: they do not elevate cholesterol and triglyceride levels. As we will see later, the fats in chocolate are harmless in other important ways too.

But the most important component of dark chocolate, and the real reason you should be making chocolate a part of your diet, is the flavonoids that turn the cocoa beans purple. Dark chocolate is absolutely loaded in a kind of flavonoid called polyphenols. The sub class of polyphenols found in chocolate is known as flavanols, or flavon-3-ols, and include catechin, epicatechin and proanthocyanidins. Dark chocolate also includes the flavonoid-like resveratrol that has become famous from red wine and the methyxanthine theobromine. Unlike the flavonoids, theobromine is not negatively affected by processing. As we'll see later, theobromine, though much less discussed than the flavonoids, may also turn out to be an important component of chocolate.

Flavonoids

Flavonoids are a group of pigments found in plants that are largely responsible for the colour of many fruits and flowers: they make cranberries, cherries and currents red; they make blueberries, blackberries and dark grapes dark purplish-blue. In the plant, they give the fruit colour; in your body, they give you health. Flavonoids are responsible for the health providing properties of many famous foods and herbs. Consider some of the foods and drinks that are so good for you largely because of the flavonoids they contain: blueberries, cranberries, citrus fruits, garlic and onions, red wine and green tea. And consider some of the best known herbs: *Ginkgo biloba*, turmeric, hawthorn berry, bilberry, grapeseed extract, milk thistle, St. John's wort and soy.

Flavonoids have a huge number of important, beneficial actions in your body: they are anti-inflammatory, anti-allergic, antiviral and anticarcinogenic. Perhaps most importantly, they are powerfully antioxidant.

Antioxidants provide your body with crucial protection from free radicals. Free radicals are terribly destructive molecules that vandalize your body. They are highly unstable because they have an unpaired electron, and they can't stand it. So, thinking only of themselves, they try to restore their stability by ripping electrons from their molecular neighbours, destroying those around them in the process and damaging your body. Free radical damage is an important cause of an astounding number of today's most serious and common diseases. Free radical damage is an important cause of the aging process and of scores of diseases, from cancer and heart disease, to cataracts, arthritis and Alzheimer's.

The most famous antioxidants are the vitamin antioxidants vitamin C, vitamin E and betacarotene. But the antioxidant activity of flavonoids, though less well-known, is much more potent and ranges much more widely.[1,2]

There are many kinds of flavonoids. Some of the best known and most important are isoflavones; citrus bioflavonoids; quercetin; and polyphenols, including the catechin, epicatechin and epicatechin gallate most famously found in green tea, and proanthocyanidins.

Isoflavones

Isoflavones are most famously found in soy. Soy isoflavones are mildly estrogenic. They are way milder than your body's own estrogen. This gives them the amazing dual ability of raising your estrogen when that is needed and lowering it when that is. If your estrogen levels are low, as in menopause, then the isoflavones from soy gently raise your estrogen level when they bind to an unoccupied estrogen receptor; when your estrogen levels are too high, as in breast cancer or uterine fibroids, then they lower your estrogen level by stealing a receptor from your body's own more powerful estrogen. This made-to-order dual ability of soy isoflavones allows them to help both the psychological[3] and the physical[4,5,6,7] symptoms of menopause--soy isoflavones work even better than hormone replacement therapy[8]—and breast cancer. Soy isoflavones have been shown to reduce the risk of developing breast cancer, the risk of recurrence of breast cancer and the risk of dying from breast cancer[9,10]. Soy isoflavones have also been shown to fight osteoporosis by increasing bone mineral density.[11,12,13,14]

Citrus Bioflavonoids

The bioflavonoids found in citrus fruits like grapefruits and oranges are antioxidants. They also increase the intracellular antioxidant vitamin C in your body. These flavonoids are particularly good at decreasing the permeability and fragility of capillaries and at reducing bruising and swelling. The effect these flavonoids have on the capillaries make them especially useful for treating varicose veins and hemorrhoids,[15,16,17,18,19,20] as well as chronic venous insufficiency.[21,22,23,24,25,26,27,28,29]

Quercetin

Quercetin is a flavonoid that is powerfully anti-inflammatory. Because it inhibits the manufacture and release of histamine, it is one of the best treatments for allergies. Quercetin is amongst the most powerful antiviral flavonoids and, along with the flavonoid curcumin, found in the herb turmeric, it is one of the most effective flavonoids against cancer.[30,31] Quercetin's cancer fighting ability is wide ranging: it is valuable for cancers of the breast, ovaries, prostate, colon, rectum, skin, lungs and brain. Quercetin is also powerfully antioxidant.

Polyphenols

Polyphenols are most famously found in green tea. They include catechin, epicaechin, epicatechin gallate and epigallocatecin gallate. The polyphenols found in green tea have greater antioxidant activity than the better known antioxidants vitamins C and E.[32] These flavonoids are important protectors against cancer: drinking green tea is one of the reasons why cancer rates are lower in Japan. And green tea is very versatile: it seems to protect against a very wide range of cancers, including oral cancers;[33] stomach cancers;[34,35] esophageal cancer;[36,37] colon, rectal and pancreatic cancers;[38,39,40,41] lung cancer;[42] breast cancer[43,44,45] and prostate cancer.[46,47]

Green tea polyphenols have also been shown to help fight heart disease, including elevated cholesterol,[48,49,50,51,52,53,54] blood pressure[54] and stroke.[55] And the polyphenols in green tea also prevent tooth decay,[56] cavities[57] and periodontal disease, including gingivitis.[58,59,60,61]

Proanthocyanidins

Proanthocyanidins are powerful antioxidants and one of the most valuable kinds of flavonoids. Proanthocyanidins are capable of antioxidant activity that is about fifty times more potent than the antioxidant activity of vitamins C and E. And these flavonoids are not only more potent, they are more versatile too. Most antioxidants work exclusively against either fat-soluble or water-soluble free radicals. Vitamin C is the primary water-soluble antioxidant, and vitamin E is the primary fat-soluble antioxidant. Proanthocyanidins have the rare flexibility to protect against both. Proanthocyanidins also increase intracellular levels of vitamin C.

Proanthocyanidins also inhibit the destruction of collagen. Combined with its anti-inflammatory properties, these affects make proanthocyanidins valuable for any type of arthritis. When you add in its power to decrease capillary fragility and permeability, you have the perfect recipe for varicose veins[62,63] and chronic venous insufficiency,[64,65,66,67] the circulatory disease of the legs that causes edema, pain, swelling, itching and cramps.

Important proanthocyanidin rich herbs include grapeseed extract, pine bark extract, bilberry, cranberry and hawthorn.

The flavonoids found in dark chocolate are the valuable and powerful antioxidant flavonoids catechin, epicatechin and proanthocyanidins. But, as you shall see, the benefits of dark chocolate flavonoids go well beyond their antioxidant activity. Much of the power of dark chocolate flavonoids derives from powers other than antioxidant.

Important Flavonoid Rich Herbs

Herb	Specialty
Ginkgo biloba	Memory and Cognition
Hawthorn	Heart
Bilberry	Eyes
Cranberry	Urinary Tract
St. John's wort	Depression
Green Tea	Cancer and Heart
Grape seed	Veins and General Antioxidant
Pine Bark	Veins and General Antioxidant
Elderberry	Cold and Flu
Garlic	Heart, Cancer, Antimicrobial, Antifungal
Turmeric	Cancer, Diabetes, Heart, Inflammation
Milk Thistle	Liver
Soy	Cancer, Heart, Menopause, Bones

PART 2:
Chocolate and Heart Health

CHAPTER 3

The Science of Valentine's Day: It's All True

Every romantic knows that chocolate is good for the heart. On Valentine's Day, chocolate is even shaped into hearts. Every year, on the most romantic of holidays, hopeful suitors and long time lovers bring gifts of chocolate hearts and chocolates packaged in heart shaped boxes.

The idea of chocolates packaged in heart shaped boxes for Valentine's Day apparently goes back to the marketing genius of Richard Cadbury who first sold his chocolates that way in the 1840's. But science is slower than marketing, and it would take researchers almost a century and a half to catch on.

In the early 1980's, a Harvard physician named Norman Hollenberg found the papers of a Doctor B.H. Kean who had worked among the indigenous Guna people on the San Blas Islands off the north coast of Panama. Dr. Kean had observed that high blood pressure was incredibly rare among the Guna people and that, surprisingly, it did not go up as they aged. He also noted their remarkably low rates of death from cardiovascular disease. When they left the island for Panama City their rates of high blood pressure caught up to the Guna of the mainland. And, as they aged, rates of high blood pressure raised too.

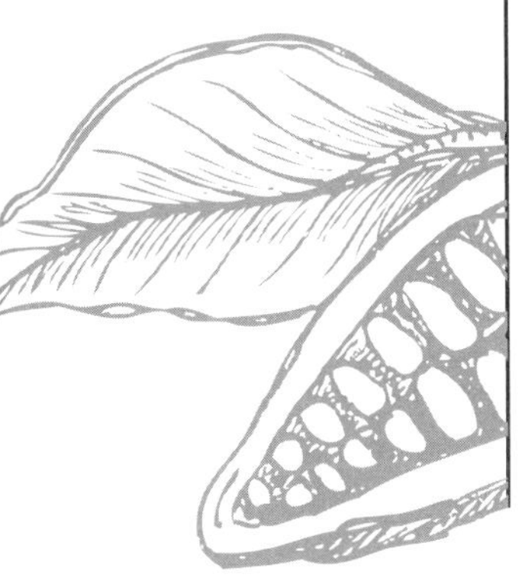

The protective factor, obviously, was not genetic. On the mainland, blood pressure rates were unremarkable; on the island, they were seemingly magically protected. The difference was diet. The traditional Guna diet featured a very natural, minimally processed, flavonoid-rich cocoa that was, apparently, consumed five times a day (that's my kind of diet!). But the multiple cups of chocolate drank by the Guna of the mainland was highly processed and low in flavonoids. And the theory was first born that flavonoids found in chocolate may protect the heart by lowering blood pressure.

A quarter of a century later, Hollenberg would team up with Naomi Fisher and other researchers and scientifically pinpoint the reason: flavanol-rich chocolate made the blood vessels dilate by increasing nitric oxide[1]. Others would soon confirm their findings[2,3] and the serious science of proving the long known Valentine's Day link between chocolate and the heart had begun.

Chocolate and the Heart

Chocolate's ability to benefit the heart is considerable. When we think of dietary changes that benefit the heart, we usually think of bad things we have to cut back on. We seldom think of delicious treats we have to increase. But eating more dark chocolate decreases your risk of getting, or dying of, several serious, common heart conditions.

Coronary Heart Disease

Coronary heart disease refers to the narrowing of the small blood vessels that supply blood and oxygen to the heart. The narrowing is caused by the buildup of plaque. If there is enough narrowing to reduce or block the flow of oxygen-rich blood to the heart, angina or a heart attack can occur. Coronary heart disease is the leading cause of death in the United States.

That means that a lot of people could benefit from eating dark chocolate. Because a 2006 meta-analysis put together the results of seven studies and found that the flavonoids in chocolate may lower the risk of dying from coronary heart disease.[4]

Since then, the evidence has mounted that dark chocolate can both prevent coronary heart disease and reduce your risk of dying from it if you do get it. When a huge study of 4,970 people between the ages of 25 and 93 compared people who ate no chocolate (we have no idea where they found them!) to people who ate chocolate between 1 and 4 times a week, they found that the chocolate eaters were 26% less likely to have coronary heart disease. When they compared them to people who ate chocolate more than 5 times a week, they found a decreased risk of a full 57% in the chocolate eaters. By the way, people who ate candies that were not made of chocolate five times a week or more had a 49% increased the risk of coronary heart disease.[5]

A study that followed 20,951 people for almost twelve years found that the ones who ate the most chocolate had 12% less risk of coronary heart disease than the ones who ate the least. The authors also did a meta-analysis of nine studies that included 157,809 people. The meta-analysis revealed that the ones who ate the most chocolate had 29% lower risk of coronary heart disease and 45% lower risk of dying from cardiovascular disease than the ones who ate the least.[6] Unfortunately, the study lumped all kinds of chocolate together: so, the results might have been even more impressive if just dark chocolate was included.

Coronary heart disease is caused by a buildup of atherosclerotic plaque. In a study of 2,217 people who had higher than expected risk of coronary heart disease, people who ate chocolate 1-3 times a month were 5% less likely to have calcium buildup in the coronary arteries causing atherosclerosis. Eating more chocolate helped even more. Eating it once a week decreased the risk by 21%, and eating chocolate 2 or more times a week decreased the risk by 31%.[7] This was the first study to show that eating chocolate protected against atherosclerosis.

Chocolate is powerful enough to protect you even if you already suffer from coronary heart disease. If you have suffered a myocardial infarction (heart attack), then eating chocolate just once a week decreases your risk of dying of coronary heart disease by 44%. And if you enjoy chocolate twice a week or more, the risk of death goes down by an even greater 66%.[8]

Cardiovascular Disease

Cardiovascular disease is a broader term that coronary heart disease that encompasses all of the diseases of the heart and circulatory system. Cardiovascular disease accounts for an astonishing 29% of all deaths in Canada and 25% of all deaths in the United States.

In 2006, researchers systematically reviewed 136 studies on the benefits of chocolate for cardiovascular disease. These early short term and population (epidemiological) studies suggested that chocolate flavonoids likely protect against cardiovascular disease. Interestingly, the studies also suggested that, although you would expect differently, even though the stearic acid in chocolate is a saturated fat, it did not increase the risk of cardiovascular disease.[9]

Later studies would continue to bear out this exciting news for chocolate lovers: eating dark chocolate actually reduces your chances of developing cardiovascular disease. A systematic review of the research identified a study that found a 35% reduced risk of cardiovascular disease for people who ate chocolate at least once a week.[10] That's a sacrifice I'd be willing to make to reduce my risk of cardiovascular disease by a third!

Similarly exciting results were found in a larger pool of subjects. When researchers combined seven observational studies into one big meta-analysis of 114,009 people, they found that when you compare the people who eat the most chocolate to the people who eat the least, a 37% reduced risk of overall cardiovascular disease is uncovered.[11] Though these studies are uncontrolled, they once again suggest that when you look at real world populations of people, the ones who enjoy the most chocolate also enjoy around a one third reduction of the risk of developing cardiovascular disease.

And, as with coronary heart disease, eating dark chocolate continues to be beneficial even if you already do have a cardiovascular disease. When researchers followed 470 elderly men for 5 years, and then followed up after 15 years, they found that the ones who ate the most cocoa were 50% less likely to die of cardiovascular disease during the 15 year follow up than the men who ate the least. And you didn't even have to eat very much to cut your risk of dying of the disease in half: the men who benefitted from that heart protection only averaged a small 4g serving of chocolate a day.[12]

Stroke

A stroke is a sudden loss of brain function caused by the interruption of blood flow to the brain or by the rupture of blood vessels in the brain. If the stroke is caused by a block of blood flow, it is called an ischemic stroke; if it is caused by the rupture of blood vessels, it is called a hemorrhagic stroke. Ischemic strokes are the most common. Either way, the stroke starves the brain of blood and oxygen, and the brain cells begin to die. Stroke is the third leading cause of death in Canada, accounting for 6% of all deaths. In the United States, stroke accounts for 5.3% of all deaths.

The good news is that one of the exciting new discoveries about dark chocolate is that it is able to reduce your chances of suffering a stroke. A study of 19,357 people found that people who eat the most chocolate are 39% less likely to suffer a stroke or a heart attack. The protection may be greatest for stroke.[13]

A study that followed 20,951 people for almost twelve years found that while 5.4% of those who ate the least chocolate suffered a stroke, only 3.1% of those who ate the most chocolate did. When the authors conducted a meta-analysis of nine studies that included 157,809 people, they found a 21% reduced risk of stroke for the people who ate the most chocolate versus the people who ate the least.[14] Unfortunately, the study lumped all kinds of chocolate together—including junky candy bars--so the results might have been even more impressive if just dark chocolate was included.

The first study to focus just on strokes was a ten year study of 33,372 Swedish women. The study concluded that each 50g per week of chocolate decreased the women's risk of stroke by 14%.[15] In the 1990's, when much of this study was conducted, about 90% of the chocolate being consumed in Sweden was milk chocolate that contained about 30% cocoa solids. It would be interesting to know if these already impressive results would have been even more impressive with dark chocolate that contained at least twice as much cocoa.

A second study also found that chocolate protects women against strokes. The large study included 38,182 men and 46,415 women between the ages of 44 and 76 and followed them for an average of 12.9 years. It found that women who eat chocolate have a significant 16% lower risk of having a stroke. Men have a 6% reduced risk of stroke, but the benefit for the men was not statistically significant.[16] The study does not seem to differentiate between eating dark chocolate or other less healthy forms of chocolate like milk chocolate. It would be interesting to see if the benefit for men would be significant if only dark chocolate was included.

The first study only looked at the effect of chocolate in women, and the second did not find a significant benefit in men. So, does chocolate have the same ability to prevent strokes in men?

To find out, the same group of researchers who conducted the women only study, looked this time at 37,000 healthy men between the ages of 45 and 79. And they found that chocolate does benefit men. The men who ate the most chocolate (62.9g a week) were less likely to suffer a stroke than men who ate no chocolate at all. Eating chocolate reduced the risk of both ischemic and hemorrhagic stroke. Altogether, eating chocolate was associated with a 17% decreased total stroke risk.[17] So, the results were very similar for men and for women.

When these researchers conducted a meta-analysis of five studies, the result was a 14%-19% reduction in the risk of a stroke when you eat about 63g of chocolate a week.[17] Again, in this meta-analysis, the type of chocolate the people ate was not specified. So, the benefits of chocolate may turn out to be even more powerful if only eating dark chocolate is considered.

The same large meta-analysis of observational studies that we looked at for cardiovascular disease found a larger 29% reduction in stroke risk for people who ate the most chocolate.[18]

Myocardial Infarction (Heart Attack)

The medical term for what is commonly known as a heart attack is a myocardial infarction. A myocardial infarction occurs when a blood clot blocks one of the coronary arteries that supply blood and oxygen to the heart. When the heart is starved of the blood and oxygen it needs, the heart cells begin to die. Every seven minutes in Canada, someone suffers a heart attack, and 16,000 people die each year as a result of one. In the U.S., someone has a heart attack every 34 seconds: that's almost three quarters of a million Americans a year having a heart attack.

Eating dark chocolate can help you to survive after a heart attack and may help to prevent heart attacks.

A study of 19,357 adults found that people who ate the most chocolate had a 39% lower risk of suffering from either a stroke or heart attack, although the protection may have been greater for stroke than heart attack.[13]

And what if you've already had a heart attack? A huge study of over a thousand people looked at what the affect was of eating chocolate on people with coronary heart disease who had survived a first heart attack. The study found that eating chocolate protected you from subsequently dying of heart disease. Over the eight year follow up period, hazard ratios went down by 27% for people who ate chocolate less than once a month, by 44% for people who ate chocolate up to once a week, and by a full 66% for people who ate chocolate at least twice a week. The researchers concluded that long term chocolate consumption is associated with a strong protective effect on subsequent cardiac mortality.[19] This study was conducted in Sweden, and, as we just saw in the stroke study of Swedish women, much of the chocolate eaten in Sweden at that time was 30% cocoa milk chocolate, so the protective effect of chocolate may be even more powerful if you eat dark chocolate.

All-Cause Mortality

And one more piece of good news. When some of these studies were looking at dark chocolate's ability to prevent death from different kinds of heart disease, they discovered an additional benefit: dark chocolate may prevent premature death from any cause.

The study of elderly men that found a 50% reduced risk of death from cardiovascular disease also found a 47% reduced risk of dying from any cause during the study.[12]

CHAPTER 4

Chocolate and Cholesterol

Cholesterol is complicated. We hear a lot about cholesterol being bad and needing to reduce our cholesterol. Well, that's both true and not true.

Just as there are good fats and bad fats and good carbohydrates and bad carbohydrates, so there are good cholesterols and bad cholesterols. Saturated fats are really bad, but unsaturated fats are really good; refined carbohydrates are really bad, but complex carbohydrates are really good. The bad cholesterol is the low-density lipoprotein cholesterol, or LDL cholesterol for short; the good cholesterol is the high-density lipoprotein, or HDL cholesterol for short. To enhance the health of your heart, you do want to decrease your levels of LDL, but you want increase your levels of HDL.

Chocolate and LDL- Cholesterol

One of the most consistent findings about dark chocolate is that it lowers levels of the dangerous LDL cholesterol. One of the first reports of this benefit was a double-blind study conducted in 2007 that gave either a cocoa powder that was rich in polyphenols or a low polyphenols cocoa powder to people with normal to mildly high cholesterol. The study lasted four weeks, and at the end, LDL cholesterol had gone down.[1]

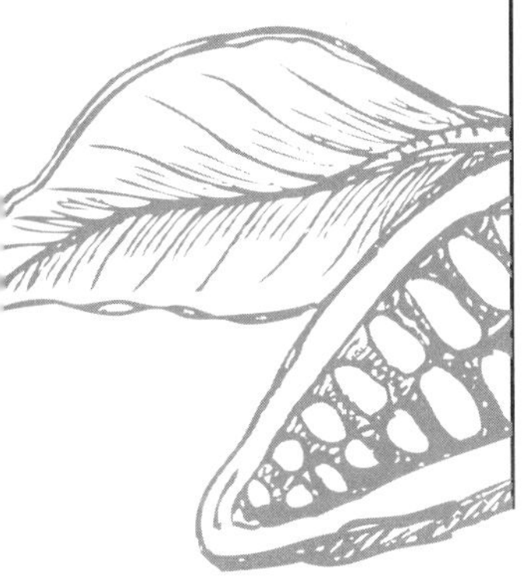

This early finding was exciting. LDL-cholesterol is an important risk factor for heart disease. Cholesterol rides around in your body on lipoproteins. These protein molecules act like shuttles for cholesterol. Low-density lipoproteins shuttle the cholesterol from your liver to your cells where they can build up and increase your risk of atherosclerosis and, eventually, of having a heart attack or stroke. For every percentage point that you manage to lower your levels of LDL cholesterol, you reduce your risk of having a heart attack by a little more than 2%.[2] So, the study suggested that eating dark chocolate rich in flavonoids could lower your risk of having a heart attack. The thought was incredible: eating chocolate could reduce your risk of heart disease.

Over the next couple of years, the early evidence continued to mount. A small pilot study of healthy people found that eating dark chocolate with 700mg of flavonoids for just one week could significantly lower LDL cholesterol by 6%.[3] That's a better than 12% reduction in the risk of a heart attack by eating chocolate.

Two other small studies found that chocolate could significantly lower LDL cholesterol in people with blood sugar problems. One was a double-blind study of people with type II diabetes who were on medication to lower their blood sugar. When they gave them either flavanol-rich cocoa or a flavanol-poor cocao (963mg of flavanols a day versus 75mg) they noticed a significant drop in their levels of LDL-cholesterol.[4] The other study compared the effect of flavanol-rich dark chocolate with white chocolate that provided no flavanols at all. The dark chocolate significantly decreased the levels of both total-cholesterol and LDL cholesterol.[5]

As the evidence for dark chocolate's beneficial effect on LDL cholesterol accumulated, researchers began to take a look at the total picture. Putting the data together for chocolate's impact on heart disease, both individual studies and a meta-analysis now showed that dark chocolate really could lower total cholesterol and the heart threatening LDL cholesterol.[6] A subsequent meta-analysis also found that chocolate significantly improved LDL cholesterol.[7]

A meta-analysis that focused specifically on studies of chocolate and cholesterol concluded that dark chocolate significantly reduces both total cholesterol and LDL cholesterol when it put together ten controlled studies.[8]

Perhaps even more importantly, when researchers put together studies on people who were actually at a high risk of cardiovascular disease, they found that, even in these more serious cases of people who really needed help, chocolate helped. The meta-analysis included 2,013 people who had high blood pressure combined with other risk factor of cardiovascular disease. It found that dark chocolate significantly lowered both total-cholesterol and LDL cholesterol.[9]

The most recent reviews have added even more evidence for the power of dark chocolate over the heart hazardous LDL cholesterol. A 2012 systematic review of all randomized, controlled studies up to the middle of 2011, for which 42 studies of 1,297 people qualified, concluded that chocolate has a significant effect on LDL cholesterol.[10] And a 2013 review concluded that cocoa reduces total cholesterol and LDL cholesterol, including reducing LDL cholesterol in people suffering from high blood pressure.[11]

This last study also found something else that is important. The review of the effect of cocoa on different risk factors for cardiovascular disease also found that dark chocolate reduces the oxidation of LDL cholesterol. Oxidation is the result of the free radical damage we discussed in chapter two. It is not unlike the oxidation that causes iron to rust. Oxidation damages LDL cholesterol and makes it damaging to the heart. This review, then, concluded that dark chocolate not only reduces the amount of LDL cholesterol but also its ability to harm you.

Several studies have found that dark chocolate has this valuable ability to prevent the oxidation of LDL cholesterol. A small, early, three week study of ten healthy people discovered that 50g of flavonoid-rich dark chocolate significantly reduced cholesterol oxidation.[12] Then a controlled study confirmed the results. Twenty-three healthy people were put either on a controlled diet or a controlled diet with the addition of 22g of cocoa powder and 16g of dark chocolate (providing 466mg of procyanidins). The dark chocolate enriched diet reduced LDL oxidation.[13]

The next step was a double-blind study. The study gave either a high-polyphenol or a low-polyphenol cocoa to 160 people for four weeks. There were three high-polyphenol cocoa groups: 13g a day, 19.5g a day and 25g a day. Oxidized LDL went down in all three of them.[14]

Most recently, a study published in 2012 found that 50g of flavonoid-rich dark chocolate is able to reduce free radical damage to LDL cholesterol in both women and men.[15]

And one more interesting possibility. A meta-analysis of the effects of flavonoid-rich cocoa on cardiovascular risk factors that found the now familiar benefit that chocolate significantly reduces LDL cholesterol also discovered the surprising finding that the effect of chocolate on cholesterol is greatest in people under fifty.[16] So, it turns out your kids are right: you should be letting them eat chocolate!

Chocolate and HDL-Cholesterol

So, chocolate offers impressive protection against heart disease by lowering both the amount of LDL cholesterol and the oxidation that makes it so dangerous. But can it also help by raising the heart healthy HDL cholesterol?

That question has been harder to answer than the perfectly consistent LDL cholesterol question. The early results were positive. In the very early days of chocolate research, a small study of healthy people found that, compared to a control diet, the same diet with dark chocolate added could increase HDL cholesterol.[17] A slightly larger study then compared dark chocolate to white chocolate and found that, while the beneficial HDL cholesterol went down by 2.9% when people ate white chocolate, it went up by a whopping 11.4% when they ate dark chocolate for only three weeks.[18]

That 11.4% increase in HDL-cholesterol was one of the most exciting chocolate discoveries yet. That's because for every percentage point you manage to raise your HDL cholesterol, you reduce your risk of having a heart attack by 3%-4%.[19] So, this early study raised the possibility that eating dark chocolate could reduce your risk of suffering a heart attack by as much as 34%-45%.

Even though you hear a lot less about raising cholesterol than you do about lowering it, raising HDL cholesterol may be even more important for preventing heart disease than lowering LDL cholesterol. Whereas, low-density lipoproteins shuttle cholesterol from your liver to your cells, where they can build up, causing atherosclerosis and increasing your risk of heart attack and stroke, high-density lipoproteins do the exact opposite: they run the return shuttle. High-density lipoproteins shuttle the cholesterol from the cells to the liver, where it is broken down and eliminated from the body. So, HDL cholesterol is preventative against atherosclerosis, heart attacks and strokes. So, an important goal of diet is to raise the heart healthy HDL cholesterol.

So, these early results for dark chocolate were exciting. Other studies continued to add to the encouraging evidence. A more reliable double-blind study had now also shown that, in people with normal to mildly elevated cholesterol, cocoa rich in polyphenols increased HDL cholesterol.[20]

A pilot study of healthy people found that eating dark chocolate significantly raised HDL cholesterol by 9%,[21] an impressive result that validated the earlier 11.4% finding.

Perhaps most importantly yet, a controlled study found that chocolate increased HDL cholesterol in people who were actually at a high risk for coronary heart disease,[22] suggesting that eating dark chocolate could help people who were really in need of help.

A small double-blind, placebo-controlled study also found that high polyphenols chocolate significantly increased HDL cholesterol levels in people with type II diabetes.[23]

But then the research took an unexpected turn. Reviews of the collection of studies began to report negative findings. A 2011 systematic review[24] included a study that found that, while dark chocolate significantly decreased both total- and LDL cholesterol, it had no effect on HDL cholesterol. The dark chocolate didn't hurt the levels of HDL cholesterol, but, unlike in the other studies, it didn't help it. It also reported a study that found that it did increase HDL cholesterol, so the results were becoming confusing. According to this review, an earlier meta-analysis found that dark chocolate does reduce total- and LDL cholesterol while having no effect on HDL cholesterol.

Then dark chocolate got hit again. Again, the bad news came out in 2011. This time the bad news came in the form of a meta-analysis that put together the data from ten controlled studies of 320 people and found, once again, that dark chocolate significantly benefits total- and LDL cholesterol but has no effect on HDL-cholesterol.[25]

Despite these anomalous 2011 studies, the weight of the research pendulum has swung back to the conclusion that dark chocolate does positively affect HDL cholesterol. It is not just that new studies are contradicting the data from 2011. The new studies are meta-analyses that are more recent analysis of the totality of the research.

Already by the end of 2011, a systematic review and meta-analysis of 24 studies had adjusted the picture by showing that flavonoid-rich cocoa both significantly decreases LDL cholesterol and significantly increases HDL cholesterol. All of the studies included in this meta-analysis were controlled studies.[26]

A year later, a meta-analysis that included only the higher quality randomized, controlled studies analyzed 42 studies that included a total of 1,297 people. It found that chocolate significantly improves levels of both LDL- and HDL cholesterol. Unlike most other studies, it also found that chocolate improved triglycerides, another kind of fat that is detrimental to the heart.[27]

Recently, a review of randomized studies has confirmed chocolate's ability to raise the levels of heart healthy HDL cholesterol while lowering total- and LDL cholesterol.[28]

A later meta-analysis that included the placebo-controlled research up to 2015, also concluded that dark chocolate flavanols significantly increase HDL cholesterol. And, again, this meta-analysis concluded that dark chocolate does significantly decrease triglycerides.[29]

And there is one more important finding about chocolate and cholesterol. A small study gave people who had either normal or moderately elevated cholesterol an amount of cocoa powder that could realistically be found in a typical diet. The cocoa was drunk in milk. Once again, the cocoa was successful in significantly increasing HDL cholesterol. But, surprisingly, it had no effect on LDL cholesterol or other cardiovascular risk factors that, as we shall see later, chocolate consistently helps. This study, along with others we will encounter as we continue to explore the research on the health benefits of chocolate, suggests that adding milk to chocolate may neutralize its superpowers: milk may be chocolate's kryptonite![30] A similar phenomenon has been identified in some of the research on tea, a beverage that contains polyphenols that are related to those found in chocolate: adding milk may cancel out the tea's benefits.

Having pointed out the similarity with green tea polyphenols, a recent study has suggested the possibility that, as valuable as the flavonoids in chocolate are, and as huge a share of the attention they get, it may be the much less discussed theobromine in chocolate, and not the flavonoids, that are the major active component that get the credit for chocolate's ability to raise HDL-cholesterol.[31]

A Comprehensive Approach to Controlling Cholesterol Naturally

It would be great if all you had to do to improve your cholesterol levels was eat dark chocolate. But, although, as we have seen, the simple, delicious step of eating dark chocolate does significantly lower total- and LDL cholesterol while raising the healthy HDL cholesterol, incorporating dark chocolate into your diet should be part of a more comprehensive natural approach to cholesterol.

Nothing is more important for controlling cholesterol than diet. What you eat is the most important determinant of what cholesterols are in your body. Luckily, eating dark chocolate lowers the bad ones and raises the good ones. But, regrettably, you have to eat more than just dark chocolate.

What chocolate has in common with all the foods that are good for cholesterol is that it grows on a plant. Plant foods contain no cholesterol. Only foods that come from animals—that is, meat, dairy and eggs—contain cholesterol. Eating animal based foods puts cholesterol into your body. But, when you eliminate animal foods from your diet, you stop putting cholesterol into your body. Animal foods are also loaded in saturated fat, and saturated fat elevates cholesterol.[32] Plant foods, on the other hand, are rich in mono- and polyunsaturated fats that actually lower cholesterol. They are also full of fiber, and fiber helps get rid of the cholesterol that is already in your body. So, animal foods contribute to your levels of dangerous cholesterol, while plant foods not only do not contribute to your cholesterol levels, they actually reduce them.

So, the most important dietary shift to make to improve cholesterol is the shift from an animal-based diet to a vegetarian diet. Vegetarians have lower cholesterol than people who eat meat,[33] and vegans have the lowest cholesterol levels of all.[34]

Fiber

There are different kinds of fiber. The one that is best for lowering cholesterol is soluble fiber. Research has identified several soluble fiber rich foods that promote healthy cholesterol levels, including oatmeal and oat bran,[35,36,37,38,39] legumes and flaxseeds.[40,41,42,43]

There are also several supplemental sources of soluble fiber that have been shown to improve cholesterol levels, including psyllium,[44,45,46,47] pectin[48] and glucomannan.[49,50,51,52]

Soy

A meta-analysis of thirty-eight placebo-controlled studies made it official: soy significantly lowers both total- and LDL cholesterol.[53] Several double-blind studies since then have added even more weight to the evidence.[54,55,56,57]

Nuts and Seeds

Think nuts are fattening? Think again! Nuts and seeds improve cholesterol and reduce your risk of heart disease. Don't believe it? A meta-analysis of twenty-five controlled studies concluded that eating nuts lowers total cholesterol by 5.1% and LDL cholesterol by 7.4%. Eating nuts was also shown to lower triglycerides. The researchers found that several different kinds of nuts were beneficial, including walnuts, almonds, hazelnuts and pistachios.[58]

Of all the cholesterol benefitting nuts, the most beneficial ones may be walnuts[59,60,61,62] and almonds.[63,64,65] But, consistent with the conclusion of the meta-analysis, hazelnuts[66] and pistachios[67] have also been shown to be effective, as have pecans. Sesame seeds and, as we have already seen, flaxseeds have also been shown to help.[68,69]

Vitamin B3, AKA Niacin, AKA Inositol Hexaniacinate

If dark chocolate and other dietary means are not enough, there are a number of effective natural supplements.

Perhaps the most effective supplement of all is niacin. Niacin lowers both LDL cholesterol and the even more dangerous lipoprotein (a), or Lp(a). Niacin also raises the healthy HDL cholesterol.

Niacin has been shown in head-to-head studies to be more effective than the cholesterol-lowering drug lovastatin. The drug lowers LDL cholesterol by 32% compared to the vitamin's 23%. But lovastatin only raises HDL-cholesterol by 7%, while niacin raises it by 33%. Remember that raising HDL-cholesterol is more important for your heart than lowering LDL cholesterol. Lp(a) is the worst cholesterol of them all, but lovastatin has absolutely no effect on it. Niacin lowers Lp(a) by a remarkable 35%.[70]

A number of other studies have confirmed niacin's superiority over pharmaceutical cholesterol fighters.[71,72,73]

A special form of niacin, called inositol hexaniacinate, does not cause the flushing that niacin can cause. It is also safer and a little more effective.[74,75,76] So, if you want to try niacin to help manage your cholesterol, look for niacin as inositol hexaniacinate.

Gugulipids

This natural cholesterol fighter comes from India. It works as well as any drug without the side effects of the drugs. Several studies have shown just how well gugulipid works.[77,78,79,80] Gugulipid can lower total cholesterol by 14%-27%, LDL cholesterol by 25%-35%, triglycerides by 22%-30% and raise HDL cholesterol by 16%-20%.

Red Yeast Rice

This one comes from China. Red yeast rice is not a well known cholesterol fighter, but it really works. Taken together, studies show that red yeast rice can lower total cholesterol by 16%-26%,

LDL cholesterol by 21%-33% and triglycerides by 20%-34%. It can raise HDL cholesterol by 14%-20%. [81,82,83,84] A massive meta-analysis of ninety-three controlled studies has testified to red yeast rice's ability to significantly lower total-cholesterol, LDL cholesterol and triglycerides while raising the HDL-cholesterol.[85]

Garlic

Garlic has been proven to benefit people who have elevated blood fats. A meta-analysis of twenty-six double-blind studies showed that garlic lowers both their total cholesterol and their triglycerides.[86] In the most comprehensive meta-analysis yet done on garlic and cholesterol, the thirty-nine placebo-controlled studies included in the meta-analysis showed that garlic significantly lowers LDL cholesterol and significantly raises HDL cholesterol.[87]

Pantethine

Pantethine, the active form of vitamin B5, is an effective cholesterol fighter.[88,89,90,91,92] It can safely lower total cholesterol by 19%, LDL cholesterol by 21% and triglycerides by 32%, while raising HDL cholesterol by 23%.

Vitamins C and E

Vitamin C lowers LDL cholesterol,[93,94] and both vitamins C and E protect LDL cholesterol from oxidative damage.[95,96]

Green Tea and Anthocyanins

Green tea contains polyphenols that are related to those found in dark chocolate. So, it is interesting to note that green tea has been shown to be able to lower total cholesterol, LDL cholesterol, the very bad VLDL cholesterol and triglycerides, while raising HDL cholesterol.[97,98,99,100]

Anthocyanins are flavonoids that are also similar to those found in chocolate. A double-blind study gave 700mg of anthocyanins or a placebo to people with high cholesterol for twenty-four weeks. Compared to the placebo, the anthocyanins lowered LDL cholesterol by 10% while raising the HGL cholesterol by 14%.[101]

Other Helpful Supplements

There are several other herbs and nutrients that can help you achieve healthy cholesterol levels. But two of the others that stand out are berberine and artichoke. Berberine has been shown to lower total cholesterol by 29%, LDL cholesterol by 25% and triglycerides by 35% in people with high cholesterol[102] and in people with diabetes.[103,104,105]

Double-blind research shows that artichoke extract lowers total cholesterol by 18.5% and LDL cholesterol by 22.9%[106] while significantly raising HDL cholesterol.[107] Artichoke can also lower triglycerides.[108]

CHAPTER 5

Chocolate and High Blood Pressure

As you remember from Chapter Three, it was the unexpected discovery that dark chocolate lowered blood pressure that led to the current excitement over chocolate as a health food and launched the modern exploration of chocolate as a health food for the heart. The observation that the Guna of the San Blas Islands received blood pressure protection from chocolate was the clue that ignited all the modern research into dark chocolate.

What is High Blood Pressure?

Your blood pressure is the measure of the pressure that builds up in your blood vessels each time your heart beats and forces blood through your arteries. High blood pressure is the result of the blood exerting too much pressure against the walls of the blood vessels, forcing your heart too work too hard to pump blood through your blood vessels.

High blood pressure is a major risk factor for heart attack, and it is the most important risk factor for stroke.

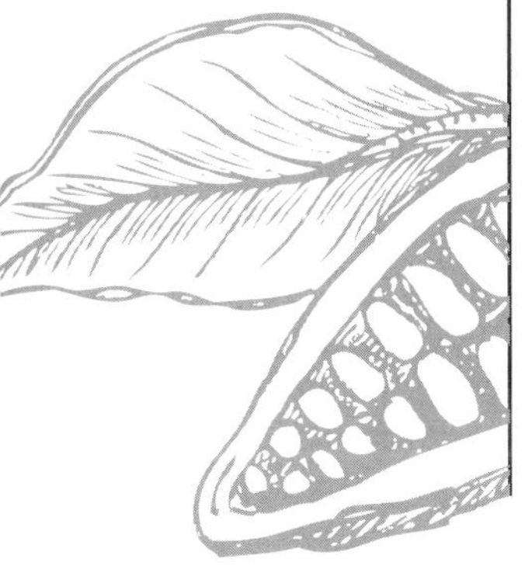

17.6% of all Canadians have high blood pressure, and 54.3% of all Americans between the ages of sixty-five and seventy-four suffer from high blood pressure.

Your blood pressure reading is expressed as two numbers: systolic blood pressure (SBP) and diastolic blood pressure (DBP). Systolic blood pressure, the first number in your blood pressure reading, is a measure of the peak reading as your heart contracts; diastolic blood pressure, the second number in your blood pressure reading, is a measure of the low reading as your heart relaxes.

A normal, healthy blood pressure reading is 120/80. If your blood pressure elevates to 140-160/95-104, it is mildly elevated. A reading of 140-180/105-114 reflects moderately high blood pressure. And your blood pressure is severely elevated if the reading is 160+/115+. If you can lower your systolic blood pressure by 4-5 mm Hg and your diastolic blood pressure by 2-3 mm Hg, it is estimated that the effect will be a reduction in your risk of cardiovascular disease and death of up to 20%.

The Research: Dark Chocolate & People with Healthy Blood Pressure

After observing the blood pressure protecting affect that dark chocolate had on the people of the San Blas Islands, researchers began to put this amazing possibility to the test.

Could something as delicious as dark chocolate really control something as serious as high blood pressure? Researchers attempted to answer this question by comparing the results on people with healthy blood pressure of eating either dark chocolate or white chocolate. Since white chocolate has no cocoa liquor and no flavonoids, it served the researchers well as a placebo. At the end of the fifteen day study, blood pressure remained healthy in both groups, but, remarkably, it really was lower in the dark chocolate group: systolic blood pressure was 113.9 in the white chocolate group but 107.5 in the dark chocolate group.[1]

And it wasn't a fluke. Another group of researchers confirmed the results: dark chocolate lowers systolic blood pressure in healthy people.[2]

And as the researchers continued to explore the effects of dark chocolate on blood pressure, the news got even better. Dark chocolate didn't just lower systolic blood pressure in people with healthy blood pressure: it lowered diastolic blood pressure too.[3]

In 2012, the highly respected Cochrane Collaboration published a meta-analysis of the research on dark chocolate and blood pressure done up until 2011. The analysis included twenty controlled studies of people with healthy blood pressure. It concluded that dark chocolate lowers systolic blood pressure by 2.77 mm HG and diastolic blood pressure by 2.20 mm Hg.[4]

The Cochrane review also suggested three other interesting things. It found that sugar free chocolate may have a greater effect than chocolate with sugar added. It also found that chocolate may have a more powerful effect on people under the age of fifty (suggesting that parents should no longer discourage their children from eating chocolate). And, interestingly, it also found that the blood pressure lowering effect of chocolate may be even greater than the research has suggested. Several studies compared high flavonol chocolate to a low flavonol chocolate control group. But the Cochrane researchers found that the low levels of flavonoids in the supposed control group may actually sometimes be sufficient to lower blood pressure. They argued that chocolate's blood pressure lowering effect may be more pronounced in studies that compare it, not to low flavonoid chocolate, but to flavonoid free chocolate.

Dark Chocolate & People with High Blood Pressure

So, what had been observed on the San Blas Islands had been confirmed by science: dark chocolate really can keep blood pressure levels healthy. But what about the important question of treatment? It had been proven that dark chocolate can keep your blood pressure low, making eating dark chocolate an important and delicious part of a strategy for preventing elevated blood pressure. But is dark chocolate's power over blood pressure great enough even to treat people who already have high blood pressure?

To answer this question, researchers gave either dark chocolate or a white chocolate placebo to people with prehypertension (130/85-139/89). Systolic and diastolic blood pressure both went down significantly in the dark chocolate group but not in the white chocolate group. The dark chocolate lowered the systolic blood pressure by 2.9 mm Hg and the diastolic blood pressure by 1.9 mm Hg. It took six weeks for dark chocolate's blood pressure lowering effect to reach levels that were statistically significant. The study's authors made the amazing conclusion that the small 6.3g amount of daily dark chocolate was comparable to comprehensive dietary modifications in its ability to lower blood pressure.[5]

These researchers made one more interesting discovery. They found that chocolate worked by increasing nitric oxide, which dilates blood vessels, which, in turn, lowers blood pressure. We'll explore this mechanism more later. But what is interesting about this discovery is that it matches the explanation of chocolate's mechanism of action that we saw Hollenberg and Fisher discover in Chapter Three.

The results seemed too good to be true. Simply eating dark chocolate could make a significant impact in people whose blood pressure was nudging up to concerning levels. But it was true. And the research continued to validate the results. A later study found a whopping 10.55 mm Hg reduction in systolic blood pressure in people with prehypertension (120-139/80-89) who ate 30g of 70% dark chocolate instead of white chocolate.[6]

Like the previous researchers, these ones found that dark chocolate significantly increased levels of nitric oxide.

So, dark chocolate works in people with healthy blood pressure. It even works in people with pre-high blood pressure. But is it powerful enough to work even in people with actual high blood pressure?

The answer is yes. When the group of people being studied included, not only people with prehypertension, but also people with actual hypertension, dark chocolate still triumphed. When the people in this study were given flavanol-rich cocoa for three months, they had a significant reduction in blood pressure.[7]

In populations of people who all had actual high blood pressure, the results were just as encouraging. One early study found a significant 5.1 mm Hg drop in systolic blood pressure and a 1.8 mm Hg drop in diastolic blood pressure in just two weeks when 100g of dark chocolate was compared to white chocolate.[8]

A number of large reviews have put all the research on dark chocolate and high blood pressure together to see just how effective a treatment dark chocolate is.

A meta-analysis of fifteen placebo-controlled studies could not detect a blood pressure lowering power of dark chocolate in people with normal blood pressure but found a substantial power in people who did have high blood pressure, or pre-high blood pressure, and actually needed it lowered. The effect was significant, lowering systolic blood pressure by 5.0 mm Hg and systolic blood pressure by 2.7 mm Hg. And the significance is not merely statistical: it is also clinical. You'll remember from the beginning of this chapter that drops in systolic blood pressure of 4-5 mm Hg and in diastolic blood pressure of 2-3 mm Hg were enough to reduce the risk of cardiovascular disease and death by up to 20%. Well, that's exactly what the authors of this study concluded. They said that the blood pressure reductions achieved simply by eating dark chocolate could translate into a 20% reduction in the risk of cardiovascular events.[9] So eating dark chocolate can reduce your risk of suffering from a cardiovascular event by 20% if you have high blood pressure!

A second meta-analysis performed the same year as this one looked at ten controlled studies of people with either pre-high blood pressure or actual high blood pressure and found that flavanol-rich cocoa significantly lowers blood pressure. These researchers found that dark chocolate reduces systolic blood pressure by 4.5 mm Hg and diastolic blood pressure by 2.5 mm Hg.[10]

A third group of researchers put together two decades of research and looked at thirteen studies of chocolate and blood pressure conducted between the years 1999 and 2011. They found that, in people with pre-high blood pressure or high blood pressure, dark chocolate drops systolic blood pressure by 3.2 mm Hg and diastolic blood pressure by 2.0 mm Hg.[11]

Even more recently, researchers conducted a meta-analysis of 2,013 people who had high blood pressure. What complicated things even more is that the people in this study had, not only high blood pressure to deal with: they had metabolic syndrome. Metabolic syndrome is a cluster of symptoms that includes three of five of high blood pressure, abdominal obesity, elevated triglycerides, low heart healthy HDL cholesterol or elevated blood glucose. Metabolic syndrome is strongly associated with dying from cardiovascular disease. So, this study was a very important test of dark chocolate.

And dark chocolate passed the test. This large meta-analysis found that dark chocolate lowers systolic blood pressure by 5.0 mm Hg and diastolic blood pressure by 2.7 mm Hg in people with high blood pressure. We met this study already in the section on cholesterol, because the study also found that dark chocolate significantly lowers triglycerides and LDL cholesterol in people at high risk of a cardiovascular event. This is important because the researchers concluded that the blood pressure and cholesterol improvements demonstrated in this study suggest that dark chocolate can reduced heart attacks and strokes by 85 per 10,000 over ten years in people at risk because of metabolic syndrome.[12]

Several other studies have also demonstrated dark chocolate's power over blood pressure.[13,14] Another meta-analysis showed dark chocolate's ability to significantly lower both systolic and diastolic blood pressure.[15] Yet another meta-analysis found that four out of the five controlled studies it looked at showed that cocoa lowered both systolic and diastolic blood pressure. The combined results showed that dark chocolate lowers systolic blood pressure by 4.7 mm Hg and diastolic blood pressure by 2.8 mm Hg, which the authors noted is not only statistically relevant, but clinically relevant in the real world.[16]

And in a strange pair of dueling reviews, a 2011 meta-analysis of twenty-four controlled studies found a significant reduction in systolic blood pressure, but not diastolic blood pressure,[17] while a 2012 meta-analysis of forty-two high quality controlled studies found a significant reduction in diastolic blood pressure and mean arterial blood pressure, but not systolic blood pressure.[18]

How Chocolate Works: The Secret Ingredient

Another meta-analysis not only reconfirmed dark chocolate's power over high blood pressure—4.1 mm Hg reductions in systolic blood pressure and 2.0 mm Hg reductions in systolic blood pressure--but shed more light on which specific component in dark chocolate may be responsible. This interesting meta-analysis of sixteen controlled studies found that dark chocolate's ability to reduce blood pressure is dependent on one of the flavanols found in the chocolate.

That flavonoids are the active ingredient in dark chocolate responsible for lowering blood pressure comes as no surprise. That's why white chocolate is used in studies as a placebo: because it has no flavanoids. That's also why the Cochrane group of researchers raised the concern over using low-flavonoid chocolate as a control: because even the small amount of flavonoids found in the supposed placebo could sometimes be enough to lower blood pressure.

But in uncovering the flavonoid that may be responsible for chocolate's blood pressure lowering effect, this meta-analysis did reveal something new, because it discovered specifically which flavonoid may be responsible. The researchers found that dark chocolate's ability to reduce blood pressure is dependent on the amount of the flavanol epicatechin that is found in the chocolate.[19]

Dark Chocolate, High Blood Pressure & Obesity

Studies have also shown the important promise of dark chocolate in lowering blood pressure in people with the additional cardiovascular burden of obesity.

Obesity is associated with high blood pressure. So, researchers conducted a small study to see what happens when obese people eat dark chocolate. The study gave 20g of dark chocolate with either 500mg or 1,000mg of polyphenols to fourteen obese people for a week. It didn't matter which dose they ate: both equally and significantly lowered their blood pressure.[20] So, contrary to conventional wisdom, it may be beneficial for overweight people to eat dark chocolate.

A second study adds even more weight to this suggestion. People who are obese or who have high blood pressure may need to be more careful when they exercise because impaired vasodilation could cause exaggerated elevations in blood pressure. So, researchers conducted a small double-blind study of twenty-one overweight exercisers. Some of them drank a high-flavanol cocoa drink containing 701mg of flavanols and some drank a cocoa drink that contained only 22mg of flavanols. The encouraging result was that the high-flavanol chocolate drink caused significantly greater vasodilation than did the low-flavanol drink: 6.1% versus only 3.4%. And the result of the superior vasodilation was that the exercise induced increase in blood pressure was reduced by the flavanol-rich chocolate drink, again showing a blood pressure benefit for dark chocolate in overweight people, specifically, this time, while exercising.[21]

Nobody's Perfect

As you can see, there have been a lot of studies of dark chocolate and blood pressure. With all the studies that have been done, the overwhelming consensus is that eating dark chocolate is an effective way to maintain healthy blood pressure and to help lower high blood pressure. To date, we can find only four studies that were unable to show a protective effect of dark chocolate on blood pressure. In science, it is rare when researchers conduct multiple studies not to have some that disagree due to different populations, poor design or any of several other reasons.

There may be several reasons why a small minority of dark chocolate studies were negative. The first negative study found no improvement in blood pressure despite the fact that it did find an improvement in the diameter of arteries.[22]

The second negative study found no effect of dark chocolate or a tomato extract when compared to a placebo in people with prehypertension.[23] However, though designed as a controlled study, the study was not fully blinded: the people in the tomato extract group didn't know if they were getting the extract or the placebo, but the people in the chocolate group were able to tell. One year later, the same group of researchers that designed this study would carry out one of the meta-analysis we looked at earlier and would find a significant blood pressure lowering effect that was impressive enough to translate into a 20% reduction in the risk of cardiovascular events.

The other two negative studies are interesting because of the information they do provide. The first found no effect on blood pressure when it delivered the chocolate in a dairy drink.[24] The final study to find no effect on blood pressure gave chocolate in milk to people with moderately high cholesterol but no high blood pressure.[25] Both of these negative studies used milk.

We saw this possible confounding effect of milk in the cholesterol chapter also. As we saw there, the final negative blood pressure study also found no effect on total cholesterol, LDL cholesterol or triglycerides, which was anomalous. Taken together, these two studies suggest the possibility that milk neutralizes the cardiovascular benefits of chocolate.

A Comprehensive Approach to Controlling Blood Pressure Naturally

Eating dark chocolate has been demonstrated to be an important and significant way of controlling blood pressure. The results are not meaningful in a merely statistical or mathematical way. They have been shown to be clinically significant in a way that could substantially lower the real life cardiovascular effects of having high blood pressure. As effective as dark chocolate is, though, it should be a part of a more comprehensive natural approach to managing high blood pressure.

Diet

Cardiovascular diseases are very amenable to dietary solutions. So, as with cholesterol, the most important first step in returning your blood pressure to healthy levels is improving your diet.

Because it is rich in potassium, magnesium, calcium, complex carbohydrates, fiber, essential fatty acids, folic acid and vitamin C, but low in saturated fat, a vegetarian diet is ideally tailored to lowering blood pressure. That's why vegetarians have lower blood pressure than people who eat meat[26,27] and lower rates of high blood pressure.[28] A vegetarian diet is not only effective at preventing high blood pressure, it is also effective at treating it.[29,30]

The DASH (Dietary Approaches to Stop Hypertension) studies have shown that diets high in fruit, vegetables, low-fat dairy, nuts, fiber, potassium, magnesium and calcium and low in cholesterol, saturated fat, total fat, sugar and meat can massively reduce blood pressure in only two weeks.[31]

Sodium & Potassium

It is well known that reducing salt is important for lowering blood pressure. Adding salt increases blood pressure;[32] reducing salt decreases blood pressure.[33,34,35] What is less well known is that at least as important as reducing your intake of salt is increasing your ratio of potassium to salt. To fully address the problem of high blood pressure, you have to have a lot more potassium in your diet than salt. But the standard North American diet provides at least twice as much salt as potassium. The fastest and most effective way to increase the ratio of potassium to salt in your diet is to switch to a vegetarian diet. Plant foods are much higher in potassium. Most meats have a potassium:sodium ratio of about 4:1 to 6:1. Most fish have a potassium:sodium ratio of only about 2:1 to 4:1. Most fruits and vegetables have a potassium:sodium ratio of at least 50:1 and many of them of over 100:1.

Minerals that Lower Blood Pressure

The most important minerals for blood pressure are potassium and magnesium. A meta-analysis of nineteen studies shows that supplementing potassium significantly lowers blood pressure.[36] A meta-analysis of twenty-two studies of magnesium found that taking magnesium is associated with a decrease of both systolic and diastolic blood pressure.[37]

Blood Pressure and the Fats You Eat

The kind of fat you feature in your diet is an important determinant of your blood pressure: saturated fat elevates your blood pressure; polyunsaturated fat lowers your blood pressure.[38,39]

One important source of omega-3 polyunsaturated fats is flax seeds and flax seed oil. When people with peripheral artery disease were given either 30g of ground flax seed or a placebo for six months, those who had high blood pressure experienced an impressive drop of 15 mm Hg in systolic blood pressure and a 7 mm Hg drop in diastolic blood pressure.[40]

Another heart healthy oil is olive oil. Olive oil is a monounsaturated fat. Double-blind research found that two to three teaspoons of olive oil a day allowed people with moderate high blood pressure to reduce their medication by 48% and still significantly lower their blood pressure.[41]

Soy and Blood Pressure

When all the double-blind studies that had been done on soy protein and blood pressure were put together into a meta-analysis, the researchers concluded that soy isoflavones significantly decrease both systolic and diastolic blood pressure. They found that, in people who actually have high blood pressure, the reductions in systolic blood pressure are actually comparable to reductions achieved with blood pressure medications.[42]

Vitamin C

Many population studies have found a correlation between higher vitamin C levels and lower blood pressure and that the more vitamin C you get in your diet, the lower your blood pressure.[43] A meta-analysis of twenty-nine studies found that supplementing vitamin C lowers systolic blood pressure by 3.84 mm Hg and diastolic blood pressure by 1.48 mm Hg. In people who had high blood pressure and actually needed to lower it, the results were even better: 4.85 mm Hg and 1.67 mm Hg.[44]

B Vitamins

A group of B vitamins, made up of folic acid, B6 and B12, is also important for treating blood pressure. B6, for example, has been shown to significantly lower blood pressure in people with high blood pressure.[45] This group of B vitamins is capable of controlling homocysteine. Homocysteine is a crucial risk factor for atherosclerosis, and atherosclerosis is a major cause of high blood pressure.

Coenzyme Q10

Another crucial nutrient is coenzyme Q10. Research shows that CoQ10 significantly lowers high blood pressure.[46,47] When people with high blood pressure were given either 60mg of CoQ10 or a placebo twice a day for twelve weeks in a double-blind study, there was a significantly greater reduction of blood pressure in the CoQ10 group.[48]

Garlic

An important herb for high blood pressure is garlic. One double-blind study of people whose high blood pressure was not being adequately controlled by blood pressure medications found that adding aged garlic extract to the meds significantly lowered their systolic blood pressure.[49] A meta-analysis of placebo-controlled studies of garlic and people with high blood pressure demonstrated that garlic reduces both systolic and diastolic blood pressure better than a placebo. According to the study's authors, the effect is comparable to blood pressure medication.[50]

Flavonoid Relatives of Chocolate

A group of flavonoids known as anthocyanins are found in berries like blueberries, cranberries, black currents and purple grapes. People who eat the most anthocyanins have 8% less risk of developing high blood pressure.[51] And blueberries have been shown to significantly lower systolic blood pressure and to significantly lower diastolic blood pressure in people who actually have high blood pressure.[52]

The closely related flavonoids known as proanthocyanidins are found in supplements like grapeseed extract and pine bark extract. Grapeseed extract has been shown to lower both systolic and diastolic blood pressure better than a placebo.[53] Double-blind research has also demonstrated the ability of pinebark extract to significantly lower blood pressure in people with mild high blood pressure.

Hawthorn and Olive Leaf Extract

The most valuable herb for heart health is hawthorn, and several studies have confirmed its ability to lower blood pressure. For high blood pressure, hawthorn works especially well when combined with olive leaf extract. Olive leaf extract is capable of significantly lowering blood pressure in people with high blood pressure.[54] In the most important study of olive leaf extract, the herb was shown to be as effective as the ACE-inhibitor captopril. Actually, the herb was better, because it reduced cholesterol and triglycerides significantly better than the drug.[55]

Hibiscus

The herb hibiscus can lower blood pressure.[56,57] People with mild to moderate high blood pressure have been shown to respond as well to a tea made from hibiscus extract that is standardized for anthocyanins as they do to the ACE-inhibitor captopril.[58]

Reishi

The Chinese medicinal mushroom reishi, is a good heart herb and has been shown in double-blind research to significantly lower blood pressure. When people with high blood pressure who did not respond to ACE inhibitors (captopril or minodipine) added reishi to their meds, their blood pressure dropped significantly.[59]

Yarrow and Other Herbs

The herb yarrow has also been shown to significantly lower blood pressure.[60]

Other helpful blood pressure herbs include mistletoe, *Coleus forskohlii* and celery seed.

When treating high blood pressure, you should also lose extra weight, exercise, quit smoking and eliminate food allergies. Acupuncture is also very helpful.

CHAPTER 6

Chocolate and The Endothelial Wall

Though high blood pressure and cholesterol problems will be much more familiar to you, one of the most crucial actions of dark chocolate is on the endothelial wall. Though much less part of the everyday conversation about cardiovascular health, a healthy endothelial wall is no less crucial.

What is an Endothelial Wall?

The endothelial wall is a single layer of cells that lines the inside of heart and blood vessels. If this vital cell wall gets damaged by free radicals, or by other causes, it becomes possible for cholesterol to deposit and for plaque to develop, eventually blocking the artery and bringing about atherosclerosis. The endothelial cell wall plays a vital role in the regulation of blood vessel tone and structure as well as vascular inflammation and clot formation. So, maintaining a healthy endothelial wall is crucial.

Dark Chocolate and the Endothelial Wall

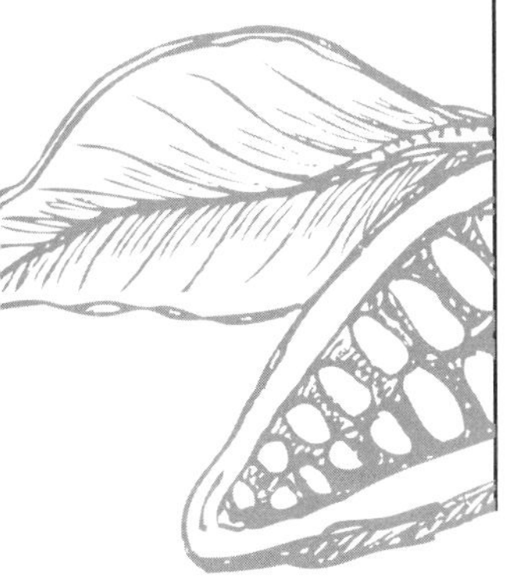

Eating dark chocolate helps this goal in two important ways. Firstly, dark chocolate acts like a call to the repairman by elevating endothelial progenitor cells in the bone marrow that help repair the damaged endothelial wall.

Secondly, the flavanols found in dark chocolate increase levels of nitric oxide. Nitric oxide is well known as the little pill people pop in the movies to prevent them from dying from heart failure. Nitric oxide is a gas that is produced by the endothelial cells that acts as a relaxing factor. It helps maintain the health of the endothelial wall and causes narrowed blood vessels to relax and expand, increasing blood flow and oxygen. Nitric oxide also improves the flexibility of the vessels.

Nitric oxide was first described in 1980, and, so important was its discovery for cardiovascular health, that, in 1998, the Nobel Prize for biology and medicine was awarded to the pharmacists who characterized its role.

You might remember the Kuna Indians of the San Blas Islands whose low rates of high blood pressure first tipped researchers off to the cardiovascular and blood pressure benefits of dark chocolate. Researchers would soon discover that what the dark chocolate beverage was doing was providing a load of flavanols that was inducing nitric oxide to dilate their blood vessels and keep their blood pressure low.[1,2,3]

Dark Chocolate & Endothelial Function in Healthy People

In 2004, researchers published the first ever study to show that eating dark chocolate could actually improve endothelial function. This important double-blind, placebo-controlled study gave either a 46g high flavonoid dark chocolate bar (containing 213mg of procyanidins and 46mg of epicatechin) or a 46g low flavonoid dark chocolate bar to twenty-one healthy adults. Plasma epicatechin concentrations improved significantly in the high flavonoid dark chocolate group but not in the low flavonoid group. And—and here was the big news—flow-mediated dilation improved in the high flavonoid group but not in the low flavonoid group: the improvement was a significant 1.33%.[4]

What does that mean? Flow-mediated dilation (FMD) is a measure of endothelial dysfunction and blood vessel function that measures blood vessel dilation in response to increased blood flow. It is especially important in people at risk for atherosclerosis or other cardiovascular diseases. FMD is an important indicator of early stage atherosclerosis. Each 1% increase in FMD translates into a 13% reduction in the risk of suffering a cardiovascular event.

That means that this study showed that eating dark chocolate produced an improvement in FMD--an improvement in blood flow-- sufficient to reduce the risk of a cardiovascular event by 17.29%.

A systematic review and meta-analysis of controlled studies found, overall, that flavonoid rich dark chocolate significantly increases FMD by an even more impressive 1.53%. However, this study again found that, as with cholesterol and high blood pressure, milk significantly impedes the beneficial effects of chocolate on FMD.[5] Another meta-analysis of foods that are rich in flavonoids has also confirmed that dark chocolate increases FMD and lowers blood pressure.[6]

Other researchers confirmed this positive effect on FMD and added more detail. These researchers were among those who had been studying the Guna Indians. Their small double-blind study found that a high flavanol cocoa drink providing 917mg of flavanols, but not a low flavanol drink with only 37mg of flavanols, significantly increased FMD and microcirculation. They also showed that the flavanols significantly elevated nitric oxide, providing important insight into how dark chocolate works.[7]

Researchers would also discover just how fast dark chocolate works: FMD increases significantly just an hour after eating dark chocolate.[8]

As we have seen, nitric oxide helps your blood vessels to relax and expand and remain young and flexible. A recent controlled trial tested these important effects by comparing a small daily treat of just 10g of dark chocolate that was at least 75% cocoa to no chocolate at all in sixty healthy people. The study lasted for one month. Even that small amount of dark chocolate had profound effects on a number of measures of arterial health. Aortic pulse wave velocity measures arterial elasticity, an important risk factor for cardiovascular disease: it improved significantly in the chocolate group. The aortic stiffness index and the augmentation index—measures of aortic and arterial stiffness—also both improved significantly. So, dark chocolate improved the stiffness and flexibility of the arteries, significantly improving vascular function. The researchers ended their paper by saying "We can suggest flavanol-containing cocoa as a promising and powerful option for cardiovascular primary prevention".[9] "Promising and powerful": they might add delicious!

In another interesting double-blind study, researchers gave eighteen healthy people a fatty drink either with flavanol rich cocoa (918mg of flavanols) or with flavanol low cocoa (a placebo 14.68mg flavanols). They used a fatty drink because when you get large amounts of fat in your blood after eating, you get quick increases in endothelial dysfunction. But drinking the dark chocolate actually prevented the endothelial dysfunction: the FMD decreased significantly less in the flavanol rich fatty drink,[10] meaning that dark chocolate can help offset the atherosclerosis causing effect of fatty foods.

Further research has also shown that dark chocolate—which is rich in polyphenols—but not a white chocolate placebo significantly improves circulation.[11,12]

And here's some really good news. Researchers wanted to see if chocolate is specifically good for older people and the negative changes that come with an aging heart. As we age, our arteries become stiffer, and we are at increased risk for high blood pressure. Their double-blind study included twenty-two people who were younger than thirty-five and twenty people who were between fifty and eighty years old. Half of the older group had either mildly elevated cholesterol or blood pressure. Everyone was given either a placebo drink or a drink that contained 450mg of cocoa flavonols twice a day for two weeks.

After two weeks, flow-mediated dilation (FMD) was significantly higher in the cocoa flavonol group than in the placebo group for younger and older people. Measures of the stiffness of the arteries and aorta improved significantly in both the younger and the older cocoa flavonol groups. Arterial stiffness and diastolic pressure improved in the older people who were drinking the cocoa flavonol drink, while there was no improvement in the placebo group. The cocoa flavonols improved diastolic blood pressure and peripheral resistance in both younger and older people, while, again, the placebo had no effect.

So, for older people, dark chocolate significantly improved blood vessel dilation, arterial stiffness, peripheral resistance and blood pressure. This study reaffirms that dark chocolate is good for the cardiovascular system for both young and old. But, intriguingly, according to the study's authors, it also shows that dark chocolate "reverses age-related burden of cardiovascular risk in healthy elderly" people. In other words, dark chocolate actually reverses the effects of aging on the cardiovascular system.[13]

It may even be possible that dark chocolate is even better than this study found. In order to make the placebo drink more like the cocoa flavonol rich chocolate drink, the researchers added theobromine into the placebo drink. But theobromine is a component of chocolate that is largely responsible for its ability to raise the heart healthy HDL cholesterol. So, the placebo may have been more than a placebo, and the chocolate may have been even better than a truer placebo.

Dark chocolate may be helping your blood vessels to relax in another important way too. Angiotensin-converting enzyme (ACE) inhibitors are drugs that help relax blood vessels and prevent the narrowing that can cause high blood pressure. They accomplish this task by inhibiting angiotensin II, which negatively affects endothelial function, platelet aggregation and blood pressure. Dark chocolate has been shown to act as an ACE inhibitor. When healthy people were given 75g of 72% dark chocolate, there was significant ACE inhibiting activity.[14]

Dark Chocolate & Endothelial Function in People with Heart Disease

Remarkably, then, dark chocolate offers protection from and prevention of atherosclerosis and cardiovascular disease. But can it help treat people who already suffer from heart disease?

The first study to ask this question said no. This six week study found no benefit of dark chocolate over a placebo for endothelial function in people with coronary artery disease.[15] However, the severity of their coronary artery disease may have been too advanced to notice a difference in only six weeks. This was the only negative study we could find on dark chocolate and endothelial function.

Later studies would find far more positive results. In one small study, people with coronary artery disease continued to take their medications but added either a low flavanol cocoa placebo drink containing only 9mg of flavanols or a high flavanol cocoa drink with 378mg of flavanols twice a day of thirty days. Blood vessel dilation improved significantly more in the dark chocolate group. FMD improved by a significant 47%. Systolic blood pressure decreased significantly. So, this study showed that dark chocolate can improve endothelial function and blood pressure even in people with coronary artery disease already being treated with drugs.

In an even more amazing study, twenty people with stage II or worse congestive heart failure were given either 40g of 70% dark chocolate or a placebo chocolate twice a day for four weeks. FMD improved significantly in the dark chocolate group compared to the placebo group, and the diameter of the brachial artery increased significantly on the dark chocolate compared to the placebo. But the reason why this study is so amazing is that, before the people in this study ate the dark chocolate, they had tried to treat their congestive heart failure with statins, but the medication had had no effect. So, the dark chocolate was able to help people with heart disease even when pharmaceutical drugs could not. The authors of this study were impressed by this "not trivial" result. They pointed out that the people in the study had advanced heart disease, drugs had not helped, the study was rigorous and double-blinded and the benefits of chocolate were significant.[17] This is an exciting study!

Dark chocolate can even help people who need heart transplants. People who have to undergo heart transplants are vulnerable to atherosclerosis because of improper vasoconstriction. But when heart transplant patients were given either 40g of 70% dark chocolate or a flavonoid free chocolate, the dark chocolate significantly improved endothelial dependent dilation of the coronary artery compared to the placebo chocolate. Platelet adhesion also decreased significantly in the dark chocolate group.[18]

Dark Chocolate & Endothelial Function in Smokers

One of the ways that smoking contributes to heart disease is by frustrating the synthesis of nitric oxide. Less nitric oxide leads to impaired endothelial function and FMD, which leads to atherosclerosis, which causes heart attacks and strokes.

Dark chocolate enhances the dilation of arteries in smokers.[19]

A small study of people with smoking related endothelial dysfunction found that a flavanol rich cocoa drink significantly increased FMD from 3.7 to 6.6 in a week. There was already a beneficial effect after just one day. The study's authors said that the effect of chocolate in reversing the endothelial dysfunction was comparable to that of pharmaceutical drugs such as statins.[20]

Another study of smokers compared a high flavanol cocoa drink with 176-185mg of flavanols with a placebo cocoa drink that provided less than 11mg of flavanols. There was a significant increase in nitric oxide and FMD in the flavanol rich chocolate group but not in the placebo chocolate group. The chocolate was able to improve blood flow in smokers by enhancing the production of nitric oxide.[21]

In yet another study, eating 40g of 70% dark chocolate was shown to improve endothelial function in a group of twenty-five smokers in two to eight hours. The researchers then compared the 40g of dark chocolate to a 40g white chocolate placebo in twenty smokers. The dark chocolate significantly improved FMD, significantly reduced blood platelet adhesion at plaque sites and significantly increased antioxidant status. The white chocolate had no effect on any of these important measures.[22] This study, once again, showed that dark chocolate is capable of significantly improving endothelial function even in smokers.

Dark Chocolate & Endothelial Function in Overweight People

The conventional wisdom and the traditional advice has always been that chocolate is fattening and should be avoided by people who are overweight or obese. We have already seen that this accepted wisdom is wrong in the case of high blood pressure. At least two studies surprised everyone by showing that eating dark chocolate is beneficial for overweight people. The same surprising result has been demonstrated for endothelial function. At least three studies have proven that dark chocolate actually improves endothelial function in obese people.

One study looked at forty-one overweight men between the ages of forty-five and seventy. The study lasted four weeks and was double-blinded. Dark chocolate increased the FMD by 1%. 1% is just a small number in other areas, but remember, in the area of FMD, a 1% increase means a 13% reduction in the risk of suffering from a cardiovascular event. So, this study found that when overweight men eat dark chocolate, they reduce their risk of cardiovascular events by 13%. It also showed that the dark chocolate decreased augmentation index—a measure of arterial stiffness—by 1%.[23]

A double-blind study of healthy, but overweight, adults showed that dark chocolate (184mg of flavanols) increased dilation of arteries by 6% and increased blood flow by 22%: both increases were significantly greater than with a low flavanol placebo chocolate. The dark chocolate also significantly decreased arterial stiffness as measured by augmentation index in women, but not in men.[24]

A placebo-controlled study of forty-five overweight adults found that a 74g dark chocolate bar significantly improved endothelial function (as measured by FMD) and blood pressure compared to a cocoa free placebo chocolate bar. And then a second phase of the study found something interesting. It compared two cocoa drinks: one was sugar free and the other had sugar. They both managed to improve endothelial function better than the placebo. But the sugar free chocolate drink was significantly more powerful than the chocolate drink with sugar. The sugar free chocolate drink also significantly decreased blood pressure, but the sugared chocolate drink could not.[25].

We have already seen that for cholesterol, blood pressure and FMD, dairy may neutralize the cardiovascular benefits of dark chocolate. This study raises the possibility that sugar may also, at least partially, neutralize the benefits of dark chocolate. Though, in the case of endothelial function, chocolate's powers may be strong enough to at least partially overwhelm the neutralizing effects of sugar.

CHAPTER 7

Chocolate and Your Heart: Putting it All Together

We have now looked at myriad studies of dark chocolate and cholesterol, dark chocolate and high blood pressure and dark chocolate, endothelial function and your veins. The way the studies are designed might make it look like chocolate isolates one cardiovascular risk factor at a time and works on it. The studies may make chocolate look like it works like a drug that targets one problem: the way a cholesterol drug targets cholesterol or a blood pressure drug targets blood pressure.

But when you eat dark chocolate, you are not taking a drug that was designed to treat one problem: you are enjoying a natural health food that is helping all these cardiovascular risk factors at once.

Look, for example, at four review studies that put all the research together and looked at multiple risk factors for cardiovascular disease.

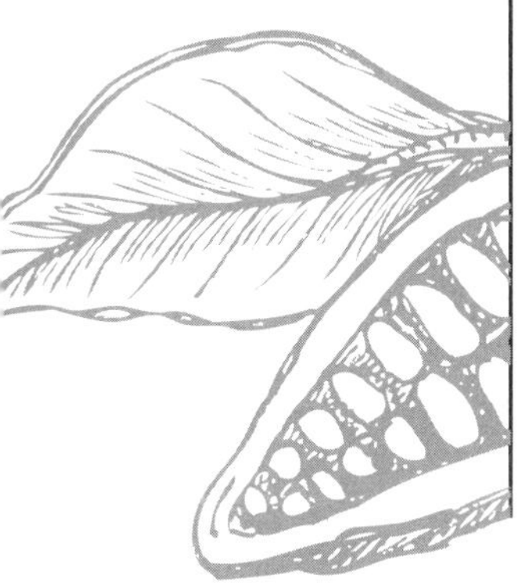

The first was published in 2011. It was a systematic review and meta-analysis of twenty-four controlled studies of flavonoid rich dark chocolate. The researchers were looking at chocolate's effect on all major risk factors for cardiovascular disease. And it found that dark chocolate benefits most of them. It significantly decreased LDL cholesterol while significantly increasing HDL cholesterol. This study detected no effect on triglycerides, though. It significantly reduced systolic blood pressure. And it found that chocolate significantly increased FMD by 1.53%.[1]

The second came one year later. This systematic review and meta-analysis was even bigger. Including forty-two studies, it confined itself to higher quality, randomized, controlled studies. It found that chocolate improved LDL and HDL cholesterol as well as triglycerides. It also found that chocolate significantly reduced diastolic blood pressure and arterial pressure. As for FMD, it detected a significant 1.3% improvement.[2]

The third was published in 2013. This review of the research found that chocolate reduces total and LDL cholesterol while increasing HDL cholesterol. It also found that chocolate has the important heart protecting effect of reducing oxidized LDL cholesterol. The review concluded that chocolate reduces high blood pressure and that it improves blood pressure and endothelial function in people who are overweight. It also revealed that chocolate often reduces inflammatory markers, including C-reactive protein, that are associated with cardiovascular disease.[3]

The fourth, and most astonishing, of the studies came out in 2014. It didn't look at risk factors, like cholesterol or high blood pressure, but at the actual diseases that result from the risk factors. The massive study had two parts. The first part followed 20,951 people for twelve years. It found that eating more chocolate was associated with lower weight, lower blood pressure and less diabetes. Compared to people who ate no chocolate, people who ate the most chocolate had 12% lower risk of coronary heart disease (angina and heart attack) and 9% lower risk of being hospitalized or dying from coronary heart disease. They had 14% lower risk of cardiovascular disease and 25% lower risk of dying from cardiovascular disease. And they had a 23% lower risk of having a stroke. Since many of the people in this study were eating milk chocolate, the results may have been even better if the study had followed only people eating dark chocolate.

The second part was a systematic review of the available research on chocolate and heart disease. It included nine studies of 157,809 people. The review concluded that eating more chocolate is associated with a significant 29% lower risk of coronary heart disease and a significant 21% lower risk of stroke. It found a significant 25% lower risk of cardiovascular disease and 45% lower risk of dying if you do have cardiovascular disease.[4]

The evidence is very convincing, then, that dark chocolate is a super food for the heart.

PART 3:

Chocolate and Diabetes

CHAPTER 8

Chocolate and Diabetes

So, now you know that chocolate is a super food. Now you're convinced, like we finally were, that chocolate is good for your heart and cardiovascular system.

But, there's no way that chocolate, the paradigm of all delicacies and sweets, could possibly be great for blood sugar. There's no way that eating chocolate could be good for diabetics. Surely, chocolate is bad for diabetes.

The unbelievably good news is that, not only is eating dark chocolate not bad for diabetes, it's good for it: it reduces the risk of developing diabetes. A systematic review and meta-analysis of seven observational studies that included 114,009 people found that, compared to people who eat the least chocolate, people who eat the most have a 31% reduced risk of diabetes. Completely against the conventional wisdom that chocolate is bad for controlling blood sugar, eating dark chocolate actually reduces your risk of diabetes by a third.[1]

What is Diabetes?

Diabetes is a chronic disease in which blood sugar levels are elevated. Most diabetics will suffer from frequent urination, excessive thirst, hunger, fatigue, weight loss and mood and vision problems. The most serious side effects of diabetes include diabetic neuropathy, or loss of nerve function, tingling, numbness and pain; increased risk of heart disease; increased risk of kidney disease; and diabetic retinopathy, an eye disease that is the leading cause of blindness.

Although diabetes is usually preventable, it is frighteningly common. In Canada 1.9 million people, or 6.5% of the population are diabetic. In the U.S., the situation is even worse: 29.1 million Americans, or an unbelievable 9.3% of the population, suffer from diabetes.

The star of blood sugar regulation is the hormone insulin. Insulin is crucial for the sugar in your blood to pass into your cells. If the pancreas cannot secrete enough insulin or the cells become insensitive to insulin, sugar cannot pass from the blood into the cells and the level of sugar in the blood becomes too high.

There are two types of diabetes. Type 1 diabetes, or insulin-dependent diabetes, usually develops in childhood. About 10% of diabetics are type 1 diabetics. In these people, the beta cells of the pancreas that manufacture insulin have been destroyed. So, type 1 diabetics do not produce enough insulin to keep blood sugar levels from rising. Type 2 diabetics, though, usually produce too much insulin. About 90% of diabetics are type 2 diabetics, and, of that 90%, about 90% of them are overweight. In these people, though there is more than enough insulin to transport the sugar from the blood into the cells, the cells have become insensitive to the insulin, producing the rise in blood sugar.

Dark Chocolate and Diabetes

Eating dark chocolate can help solve the problem of the cells' insensitivity to insulin. 100 grams of dark chocolate with 500mg of polyphenols significantly lowers insulin resistance and significantly improves insulin sensitivity in healthy people compared to a white chocolate placebo that has no polyphenols.[2] It should now not be a surprise that the people in this study who got the dark chocolate also had significantly lower blood pressure than the people who ate the white chocolate.

Dark chocolate's ability to address insulin resistance has not been seen in only one study. A meta-analysis of higher quality, controlled studies showed that dark chocolate positively affects insulin levels and significantly reduces insulin resistance.[3] A second meta-analysis of controlled studies also found that dark chocolate benefits insulin resistance. This systematic review and meta-analysis of controlled studies of flavonoid rich cocoa found that chocolate reduced HOMA-IR, a measure of insulin resistance, by a significant .94 points and increased the insulin sensitivity index (ISI) by a significant 4.95 points.[4] When a meta-analysis looked at 19 placebo-controlled studies of cocoa flavanols that were published up to 2015, it found that dark chocolate significantly decreased fasting insulin levels compared to placebo. Dark chocolate also significantly improved insulin sensitivity as measured by HOMA-IR, QUICKI and the insulin sensitivity index.[5]

So, dark chocolate can help prevent and treat diabetes by allowing more sugar to pass out of the blood and into the cells by significantly decreasing insulin resistance and improving insulin sensitivity.

Two other interesting studies also found that dark chocolate can improve insulin sensitivity. These studies are intriguing because they found something else too. Both studies once again found that dark chocolate that is rich in flavanols significantly decreases blood sugar by improving insulin resistance. But these two studies also found something else that was exciting: dark chocolate improved cognitive functioning, and the improvement in mental functioning was mainly caused by the improvement in insulin sensitivity.[6,7] We'll explore dark chocolate's exciting effect on the brain more in the next chapter. For now, what is important about these studies is that they, once again, show dark chocolate's benefit for preventing and treating diabetes and that that beneficial effect on blood sugar leads to even further exciting benefits.

Dark Chocolate & the Complications of Diabetes

As the two cognition studies show, blood sugar problems can cause complications that cascade beyond diabetes. One of the most serious complications of diabetes is the increased risk of heart disease. So, supplements or foods that benefit diabetes and, at the same time, prevent or treat the risk factors for heart disease are especially valuable. As we have already seen, chocolate has that special ability.

Sweets have always been off limits for diabetics, and chocolate has always gotten caught up in that nutritional net. But when type 2 diabetics were given 45g of 85% high polyphenol chocolate a day for eight weeks, their heart healthy HDL cholesterol went up significantly and the ratio of total cholesterol to HDL cholesterol went down significantly. There was no improvement in the placebo group.

That dark chocolate improves cholesterol is no longer a surprise: in Chapter Four, we saw tons of studies proving that chocolate benefits cholesterol. What is important about this study is that it shows that chocolate is a safe way even for diabetics to improve their cholesterol: which is very important for diabetics. In this study, dark chocolate improved their cholesterol without changing their ability to control their blood sugar. Eating dark chocolate did no harm to their insulin resistance or glycemic control, showing that the advice for diabetics to avoid sweets does not apply to dark chocolate. Chocolate safely reduces cardiovascular risk in diabetics without worsening their diabetes.[8]

So, diabetics can reduce their risk of heart disease and get the luxury of chocolate back in their lives. It may even make it easier to follow a healthy diabetes diet, free of sweets, if you are allowed to love chocolate once again. A double-blind study of one-hundred type 2 diabetics again found that chocolate can reduce the risk of heart disease and diabetes. For six weeks, the people in this study drank either 10g of cocoa powder mixed with 10g of dried milk powder in boiling water or just the milk powder in boiling water. The chocolate decreased total cholesterol by 16.5% versus 5.08% in the control group. LDL cholesterol went down by 17.54% in the chocolate group but only by 2.57% in the control group. HDL cholesterol increased by 7.58% in the chocolate group compared to 4.57% in the control group. And triglycerides went down by 13.3% in the chocolate group but by only 3.99% in the milk only group.

We have already seen that milk can impede the cholesterol and cardiovascular benefits of dark chocolate. The authors of this study acknowledged that the milk they dissolved the chocolate in could have detrimentally affected the results. Since they knew this, it is not clear why they included milk in their chocolate. A better form of dark chocolate may have produced even better results.

Free radical damage and inflammatory markers are also risk factors for diabetes, and, in this study, the dark chocolate also significantly decreased markers of inflammation. And while free radical damage increased by a significant 17.75% in the milk group, the dark chocolate prevented any significant rise in free radical damage.

The authors of this study concluded that dark chocolate may be "an exciting new area of research especially as a cardiovascular damage protective agent in diabetes patients".[9]

And chocolate exerts all of its heart protecting properties on diabetics: not just improving blood fats. A double-blind study of type II diabetics found that chocolate improves flow mediated dilation (FMD) as well as cholesterol. The study compared a flavanol rich cocoa (321mg flavanols) to a flavanol poor cocoa (25 mg flavanols). When the people in the study took the chocolate three times a day, the flavanol rich chocolate increased FMD by a significant 30% and significantly lowered LDL cholesterol. The authors of the study were impressed by chocolate's ability to improve endothelial function in diabetics and reverse their vascular dysfunction.[10]

Chocolate's powers are fast acting: they prevent some of the sudden acute effects of eating sugar. One of the reasons why diabetics have a higher risk of heart disease is that high blood sugar causes inflammation that can aggravate endothelial dysfunction and free radical damage. But when type II diabetics who were obese ate either 13.5g of high (3.5%) polyphenol chocolate or 13.5g of low (.9%) polyphenol chocolate before being given an oral glucose load, endothelial function was significantly better in the high polyphenol group and measures of free radical damage were significantly lower.[11] The long term benefits of chocolate were already known, but this was the first time science had shown that dark chocolate can even protect against the acute effects of high blood sugar on risk factors for heart disease.

Since we have already seen that dark chocolate improves insulin resistance and sensitivity and that it improves cardiovascular health, it should not come as a surprise that a number of studies have shown, not only that dark chocolate improves heart health in diabetics without harming their blood sugar control, but that it benefits both the diabetes and the heart simultaneously.

In a study of people with high blood pressure, people ate either a 100g dark chocolate bar with 88mg of flavanols or a control white chocolate bar with none. The people who got the dark chocolate bar were not only lucky because . . . well, they got the dark chocolate bar, but because they had significant decreases in HOMA-IR, which measures insulin resistance; significant increases in QUICKI, which measures insulin sensitivity; and significantly improved FMD, LDL cholesterol and blood pressure,[12] meaning that the dark chocolate improved measures of blood sugar control and cardiovascular health.

When a similar study was done on healthy people, the results were similar. HOMA-IR and QUICKI were significantly better in the dark chocolate group than in the white chocolate group and, though blood pressure was already normal in both groups, it was better in the dark chocolate group.[13]

A study that looked at sixty people who had type 2 diabetes also found simultaneous benefits for their diabetes and their heart health. Each person was given either a 25g 83% dark chocolate bar containing 450mg of flavonoids or a white chocolate bar with no flavonoids each day for eight weeks. Compared to the placebo white chocolate bar, eating the daily dark chocolate bar led to significant improvements in blood pressure and fasting blood glucose. Diastolic blood pressure went down by 5.93mm Hg but by only 1.07mm Hg in the white chocolate group; systolic blood pressure went down by 6.4mm Hg in the dark chocolate group but continued to climb by 0.17mm Hg in the white chocolate group. Eating dark chocolate led to a fasting blood glucose drop of 7.84mg/dL, while it continued to get worse by 4.0mg/dL in the white chocolate group.[14]

In the section on Chocolate and Diabetes, we looked at a meta-analysis of 42 higher quality, controlled studies that found that chocolate significantly reduced insulin resistance and improved insulin levels. What we didn't tell you then was that the meta-analysis also found that at the same time as the chocolate was benefitting blood sugar, it was also benefitting the heart. Chocolate improved LDL and HDL cholesterol and triglycerides, significantly reduced diastolic blood pressure and improved FMD by 1.3%. Remember that each 1% increase in FMD lowers the risk of a stroke or heart attack by 13%. So, chocolate reduces the risk of heart attack or stroke by 16.9%.[15]

A meta-analysis of studies looked at the effect of chocolate on people with high blood pressure and metabolic syndrome. A person has metabolic syndrome if she has any three of the following five symptoms: abdominal obesity, elevated triglycerides, low HDL cholesterol, high blood pressure and elevated blood glucose. The results showed that dark chocolate lowers both systolic and diastolic blood pressure and that it significantly lowers total and LDL cholesterol in people who are at a high risk of a cardiovascular event. The researchers said that these blood pressure and cholesterol improvements mean that 100g of dark chocolate a day can reduce cardiovascular events by 85 per 10,000 over ten years in people with metabolic syndrome.[16]

A small, but very interesting, study looked at the effect of chocolate on people with impaired glucose tolerance and high blood pressure. It found that dark chocolate, but not a placebo white chocolate, significantly decreased both systolic and diastolic blood pressure, significantly improved FMD and significantly lowered total and LDL cholesterol. It also found that the dark chocolate decreased insulin resistance and increased insulin sensitivity. None of this is new. But what is new about this study that makes it so interesting is that it is the only study that also found that dark chocolate actually increases beta cell function, the cells in the pancreas that produce insulin.[17] The ability to improve beta cell function suggests the possibility that dark chocolate could even be of some benefit to type 1 diabetics.

Dark Chocolate, Diabetes & Obesity

As we have seen in earlier chapters, dark chocolate benefits people who are overweight in a number of ways, including improving blood pressure and endothelial function. Being overweight is also a major risk factor for type II diabetes.

So, can eating dark chocolate have blood sugar balancing benefits for overweight people? When obese people who were otherwise healthy were given 20g of dark chocolate with either 500mg or 1000mg of polyphenols for two weeks, both doses significantly decreased both blood glucose levels and systolic and diastolic blood pressure.[18]

So, even if your weight is putting you at greater risk of high blood pressure and diabetes, you can go ahead and enjoy some dark chocolate each day.

A Comprehensive Approach to Managing Diabetes Naturally

The most important step in managing diabetes is eating lots of dark chocolate. Just kidding (it's the second most important step!).

The most cruelly kept secret about diabetes is that it can be prevented and treated by natural means, usually without drugs or insulin.

The most important step in preventing and treating diabetes, as with every other condition we have looked at in this book, is diet. As all the chocolate research highlights, what you eat has a major impact on your blood sugar control and on your risk of diabetes.

Ground breaking recent research has shown that you can dramatically take control of your risk of diabetes. The most important risk factors for diabetes are in your control, not in your genes. An important study asked 577 people with prediabetic impaired glucose tolerance to either take control of their diet, their exercise, both or neither for six years. These people were on their way to diabetes, but didn't yet have it. After six years, the ones who took control had 51% lower incidence of diabetes. After twenty years, they still had a whopping 43% lower risk.[19]

What are the most important ways you can take control?

Diet

The most important things you can control in your diet are fiber and fat. A high fiber diet lowers glucose levels better than the American Diabetic Association diet and as well as drugs:[20] that's another of the most cruelly kept secrets. Increase your fiber by eating whole grains, complex carbohydrates and other high fiber plant foods; don't eat refined carbohydrates, simple sugars and processed foods.

Several fiber supplements have also been shown to help: including psyllium,[21,22,23,24] guar gum,[25] pectin[26] and oat bran.[27]

As important as fiber is fat. Eating the right type of fat is crucial for preventing diabetes. What fats you eat determines what fats your cells' membranes are made of. If you eat lots of saturated fat, then it is saturated fat that your cell membranes will be made of. But if cell membranes are made up of too much saturated fat, and not enough of the polyunsaturated essential fatty acids, they lose their fluidity. When that happens, they become insensitive to insulin and the development of diabetes has begun. That's why tons of studies show that omega-3 fatty acids and monounsaturated fats protect against diabetes and saturated fats contribute to causing it.

Given that fiber and essential fatty acids are good for diabetes and saturated fat is bad for it, it is not surprising that research shows that a vegan diet improves blood sugar control in diabetics. What may be surprising is that the study found that the vegan diet is more effective than the diet recommended by the American Dietetic Association and as effective as drugs.[28] The American Dietetic Association (now known as the Academy of Nutrition & Dietetics) now admits that their evidence based review shows that a vegetarian diet lowers the risk of diabetes.

Conversely, a huge four year study showed that meat increases the risk of diabetes. People who increased their red meat by only half a serving a day increased their risk of diabetes by 48%; those who deceased it by half a serving a day decreased their risk of diabetes by 14%.[29]

Certain plant foods are especially beneficial for diabetes. Contrary to the common misconception, you should not only eat plenty of vegetables, but plenty of fresh fruit as well, including as wide a variety as possible.[30,31]

Eat plenty of nuts, seeds, legumes, garlic and onion. People who eat more whole grains, fruits, nuts, seeds, green leafy vegetables and low fat dairy are 15% less likely to get diabetes.[32] Eating two or more servings of walnuts a week reduces the risk of type 2 diabetes by 24%.[33]

Since we have already seen that the flavonoids in chocolate fight diabetes, it should not surprise you that research shows that flavonoids prevent diabetes. A large study that followed over 200,000 people for twenty-three years found that people who get the most anthocyanin flavonoids in their diet (like those found in blueberries) were 15% less likely to develop type 2 diabetes. It found that eating a lot of blueberries, apples or pears reduced the risk of diabetes by 23%.[34] And a huge meta-analysis of four studies has shown that people who have the most flavonoids in their diet are 9% less likely to develop type 2 diabetes.[35]

The flavonoids found in fruit are not the only relatives of the chocolate flavonoids to fight diabetes. The polyphenols found in green tea are also close relatives of the antioxidants found in chocolate. A large meta-analysis of seventeen controlled studies of a variety of people—including some who were of healthy weight, some who were overweight, some who were prediabetic and some who were already diabetic—found that green tea significantly reduced glucose and insulin levels. The green tea also lowered HbA1c, which is the best measure of long term blood sugar and diabetes control.[36]

Vitamins & Minerals

The most important nutrient for diabetes is chromium. Without chromium, insulin can't transport sugar from the blood into the cells, so blood sugar goes up. Chromium is well proven to help diabetes.[37,38,39] Chromium can even help type 1 diabetics. When type I diabetics were given 200mcg of chromium a day, 71% of them were able to decrease their insulin by 30%.[40]

In probably the most important study on chromium to date, type II diabetics who were already on the diabetes drug glipizide were also put on either 500 mcg of chromium or a placebo twice a day for ten months. The chromium significantly improved insulin sensitivity compared to the placebo and also led to less weight gain and less diabetes-caused tissue damage.[41]

When overweight people whose meds were failing to control their diabetes added 600mcg of chromium and 2mg of biotin in a placebo-controlled study, their blood glucose dropped a significant additional 6% and their HbA1c improved significantly.[42]

Deficiencies in the mineral zinc contribute to the development of diabetes.[43] Zinc lowers blood sugar levels even in type 1 diabetics.[44]

People with the highest blood levels of vitamin C are 62% less likely to become diabetic than those with the lowest.[45] And when type 2 diabetics add just vitamin C to their metformin, blood glucose levels and HbA1c improve.[46]

When people who are at risk of diabetes take just 365mg of magnesium a day, their blood sugar levels improve significantly.[47] Some studies show that magnesium reduces insulin requirements in type 1 diabetics[48] and that it improves insulin production in elderly type 2 diabetics.[49]

Lower levels of vitamin D are associated with insulin resistance and less ability of the pancreas to secrete insulin.[50] So, vitamin D may improve blood sugar levels and help prevent diabetes. Low levels of vitamin D increase your risk of type 2 diabetes; high levels reduce it. Research offers the hope that vitamin D may help prevent type 1 diabetes too.[51,52] Regular supplementation of vitamin D can reduce the risk of type 1 diabetes by 80%.[53]

Coenzyme Q10 improves blood glucose and insulin synthesis.[54] And lipoic acid, which significantly improves insulin sensitivity[55] is the most important nutrient for diabetic neuropathy.

Herbs

One of the most exciting herbs for diabetes is cinnamon: because of all the research, because it is simple and safe and you can cook with it and because it goes great with chocolate! There had been stories about cinnamon, but the real research began around the same time as the research on chocolate when a placebo-controlled study found that 1-6g of cinnamon reduced serum glucose in type 2 diabetics.[56] Later double-blind research would confirm that 360mg of cinnamon extract significantly improved blood glucose and HbA1c in type 2 diabetics who were already being treated with the diabetes drug gliclazide.[57] Other studies would also find that cinnamon reduces blood sugar.[58,59] Two meta-analyses of the controlled research on cinnamon have shown that its reduction in blood glucose is comparable to the diabetes drug metformin and that it significantly reduces HbA1c when it is taken as a capsule.[60,61]

Another herb that is often used in cooking that is good for diabetes is fenugreek, which has been shown to help both type 1 and type 2 diabetics. 50g of defatted fenugreek seed powder twice a day significantly lowered blood glucose compared to a placebo and also improved glucose tolerance in type 1 diabetics.[62] 15-25g of powdered fenugreek seed has also been shown to significantly lower blood sugar.[63,64] When type 2 diabetics not successfully managed by the drug sulfonylureas added either fenugreek saponins or a placebo, there was a significant drop in blood sugar levels, symptom scores and other important markers of diabetes in the fenugreek group compared to the placebo group.[65]

Garlic is yet another culinary herb that is beneficial for diabetes. Double-blind research has shown that adding 300mg of supplemental garlic three times a day to the drug metformin significantly drops blood sugar by 3.12%. When a placebo was added to the drug instead, the drop was only 1.78%.[66]

When we were in a traditional Mayan village in Guatemala, we found dark chocolate with ginger in it. Dark chocolate and ginger make, not only a great taste pairing, but a great diabetes pairing. When type 2 diabetics who are already on medication add 3g of ginger, the ginger improves serum glucose, insulin, insulin resistance, HbA1C, measures of free radical damage and inflammation significantly better than a placebo.[67]

Bitter melon has a long tradition of use for diabetes. One of its components has been shown to lower blood sugar like insulin without the side effects of insulin. When type 2 diabetics were given 100ml of fresh bitter melon, 73% of them improved significantly.[68] And 100ml of bitter melon extract has been shown to drop blood sugar by 54% in three weeks.[69]

The herb ***Gymnema sylvestre*** has the exciting ability to regenerate beta cells in type 1 diabetics. Gymnema lowers insulin requirements by 50% in type 1 diabetics. It also lowers blood sugar and improves blood sugar control.[70] Type 2 diabetics who add ***gymnema*** to their medication also have significant improvement in blood sugar control.[71]

An emerging treatment for diabetes is berberine, the active ingredient in herbs like goldenseal. 500mg of berberine taken three times a day is as effective as the drug metformin at improving blood sugar, HbA1c and insulin, with the advantage that it also lowers cholesterol and triglycerides. When drugs are not successfully managing type 2 diabetes, adding berberine significantly improves blood sugar, HbA1c, cholesterol and triglycerides.[72] Berberine has been shown to be as effective as the drugs metformin and rosiglitazone for managing type 2 diabetes.[73]

We have already seen that when people eat a lot of the anthocyanin flavonoids that are related to the flavonoids in chocolate, they reduce the risk of diabetes. Taking anthocyanin supplements also works. A double-blind study found that 160mg of anthocyanins taken twice a day reduces blood sugar and insulin resistance in diabetics.[74]

PART 4:

Chocolate and Your Mind

CHAPTER 9

Chocolate, Cognition & Mood

Eating dark chocolate has always made the two of us happy! And now scientific research is beginning to say that it really does.

The research on how chocolate affects your mind is newer and scarcer than the research on how it affects your body by benefiting your cardiovascular system and blood sugar control. But it is beginning to mount. There is good evidence that dark chocolate improves cognition and early evidence that it improves mood.

Chocolate Makes You Smarter

It seems too good to be true. Dark chocolate, it turns out, is brain food. The world just keeps getting better! Eating chocolate not only makes you healthier, it makes you smarter. A growing body of evidence is suggesting that dark chocolate improves cognition in some of the same ways it improves heart health and, surprisingly, diabetes.

We already saw in Chapter Three that dark chocolate can prevent ischemic strokes by improving blood flow to the brain. But improving blood flow to the brain also improves the brain: it improves thinking and memory.

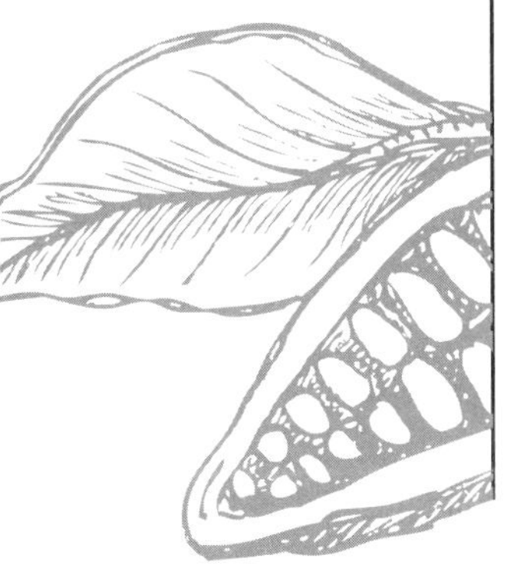

One of the first cognition studies to include chocolate was a large study of 2,031 people between the ages of seventy and seventy-four. It found that people who ate the most flavonoid containing foods had significantly better scores on tests of cognition. The study looked at chocolate, wine and tea. People who ate and drank all three had the best scores. Drinking 15-100ml of wine a day had the greatest effect; eating 10g of chocolate a day was a very close second. The researchers said, though, that chocolate's effect on cognition is probably greater because the study didn't consider what kind of chocolate was being eaten. Chocolate was effective even though much of the chocolate was probably milk chocolate. Had they been able to look at just dark chocolate, with its much greater level of active flavonoids, the chocolate would likely have improved cognition even more.[1] 10g is also a small serving of chocolate.

In another study of chocolate and cognition, 531 healthy people over the age of sixty-five were followed for four years while their dietary habits were tracked. At the beginning and end of the study, each senior took the Mini-Mental State Examination (MMSE), a measure of global cognitive function. Eating chocolate was associated with a 41% lower risk of cognitive decline, as long as they consumed less than 75mg of caffeine a day.[2]

Chocolate improves the workings of the brain in the same way it prevents ischemic strokes: it improves blood flow to the brain. Too little blood flow to the brain, known as cerebral ischemia, causes cognitive decline. When twenty-one healthy people between the ages of fifty-nine and eighty-three were given either 900mg of cocoa flavanols or a placebo with only 36mg flavanols each day for a week in a double-blind study, significantly more people in the real chocolate group had their blood flow velocity to the brain increase. The authors concluded that this result "suggests a promising role" for regularly eating cocoa in the treatment of cerebrovascular ischemic syndromes, including both strokes and dementia, because chocolate increases blood flow to the brain. Dark chocolate, it was beginning to seem, could help prevent dementia.[3]

But does increasing blood flow to the brain by eating dark chocolate really make you smarter? It does. A controlled study of thirty-seven healthy people between the ages of fifty and sixty-nine compared cocoa containing 900mg of flavanols daily to a placebo cocoa with only 10mg of flavanols. The study lasted for three months. The real chocolate improved blood flow to the dentate gyrus region of the brain and that enhanced its functioning. The functioning of the dentate gyrus region of the brain declines in old age, which is believed to be a possible cause of age-related memory decline. But the seniors who were getting the real chocolate in this study reversed their age-related memory decline: they had about a 25% increase in memory function compared to the people getting the placebo. The seniors who were getting the real chocolate performed way faster in a delayed-recognition memory test. But here's the amazing part. The researchers said that "If a participant had the memory of a typical 60-year-old at the beginning of the study, after three months that person on average had the memory of a typical 30 or 40-year-old.[4] Dark chocolate can make a senior's memory young again.

But dark chocolate can make an already young memory stronger too. So, don't worry, kids: you can eat dark chocolate too. A study of thirty healthy college students gave some of them 35g of dark chocolate (containing 773mg of cocoa flavanols) and some of them 35g of a white chocolate placebo. Two hours later, they took visual and thinking tests. The ones who got to eat the dark chocolate performed significantly better on tests of spatial memory—they got 3.6% more correct answers (and remember, they were already healthy)—and reaction time. They also performed significantly better on tests of contrast sensitivity (a full 13.3% better) and visual motion detection. So dark chocolate improved brain function and visual performance even in young students with already healthy memory and vision. The researchers believe that the improvement is because of improved blood flow to the retina and the brain.[5] Since contrast sensitivity is often weakened in older people, dark chocolate could also help them with tasks like driving.

How Does It Do It?

How can eating dark chocolate possibly make you smarter? We have already seen that one way that it helps the brain is the same way that it helps the heart: by increasing blood flow. But, it turns out, dark chocolate is doing much more than that. It is not only helping the brain the same way it helps the heart, it is also helping the brain in the same way that it helps diabetes.

An intriguing double-blind study gave ninety elderly people three different chocolate drinks. The first was high in the flavanols that are responsible for much of chocolate's health giving powers. This chocolate drink had 993mg of flavanols per serving. The intermediate flavanol drink had 520mg of flavanols, and the low dose placebo drink had only 48mg of flavanols. The study lasted eight weeks.

The people who got more chocolate flavanols did better on tests of cognition. Trail Marking Tests A and B are important tests that measure visual search speed, processing speed, mental flexibility and executive function. The time taken to complete test A decreased by 8.6 seconds and the time taken to complete test B decreased by 16.5 seconds in the high flavanol chocolate group. In the intermediate flavanol group, the times decreased by 6.7 and 14.2 seconds. Both of these improvements were significantly better than in the low flavanol group who had no significant improvement. Improvements in the Verbal Fluency Test were also significantly better in the high flavanol group than in the intermediate or low flavanol groups. This test assesses cognitive impairment in conditions like ADHD and Alzheimer's Disease.

Importantly, overall, cognitive function improved significantly in the high and intermediate flavanol groups but not in the low dose placebo group.

The researchers concluded that dark chocolate can improve cognitive performance in elderly people and that eating dark chocolate can play an effective role in countering the cognitive changes associated with aging.

But the researchers found something else. Although they found that chocolate's antioxidant and blood pressure lowering powers were partly responsible for the improvement in cognition, they found that dark chocolate's ability to improve insulin resistance was the main contributor to cognitive enhancement. That means that one of the main ways dark chocolate benefits the brain is the same way it benefits blood sugar control and diabetes.[6]

Dark Chocolate & Mild Cognitive Impairment

The authors of the study we just looked at said that their results suggest that eating dark chocolate regularly can improve cognitive performance in elderly people who do not have cognitive dysfunction. They went on to say that their findings "provide encouraging evidence" that eating dark chocolate "may be an effective dietary approach for counteracting cognitive changes associated with brain aging and offer a possible complementary strategy to support cognitive and cardiovascular health with age."

But what about elderly people who do have some cognitive dysfunction? Can chocolate still help when the changes associated with brain aging begin to impair cognition?

Mild Cognitive Impairment (MCI) is a newly recognized condition that affects as many as 42% of seniors. People with MCI may have some difficulty with memory, thinking, language and judgement, but the trouble is not debilitating enough to cause the real problems of Alzheimer's Disease. Not everyone with MCI will develop dementia, but MCI is associated with an increase in risk.

Unfortunately, research has found that drugs don't help MCI.[7] But chocolate does!

A double-blind study gave ninety people with MCI a chocolate drink containing 900mg of flavanols (high flavanol), 520mg of flavanoids (intermediate flavanol) or 45mg of flavanols (low flavanol) for eight weeks. On two tests of cognition, the high flavanol and intermediate flavanol groups improved significantly, while the low flavanol group did not. Composite cognitive scores improved in the high and intermediate flavanol groups but not the low flavanol group. The researchers concluded that flavanols found in dark chocolate benefit people with MCI, especially processing speed, executive function, language and working memory.[8] This is the first ever study of chocolate and cognitive performance in people with MCI.

Natural Treatments for
Mild Cognitive Impairment

Dark Chocolate
Ginkgo Biloba
Green Tea
Blueberries
Folic Acid, B6 & B12

Don't Worry; Be Happy! Chocolate Relaxes You and Improves Your Mood

Dark chocolate doesn't just make your thoughts and memories stronger, it makes them happier and calmer.

Emerging research is suggesting that dark chocolate affects mood. It seems that chocolate can elevate mood and reduce stress and anxiety.

The first study to discover the possible mood enhancing effects of chocolate showed that simply eating a piece of chocolate improves negative moods in the short term. It didn't seem to have much effect on neutral or positive moods, but it did improve negative mood compared to a placebo. When the researchers compared the results of a good tasting chocolate to a not good tasting chocolate (we're not sure what that is—we're yet to discover a not good tasting chocolate: the researchers called it "unpalatable" chocolate), they found that negative mood was improved after eating the tasty chocolate compared to the not good tasting chocolate. So, they concluded that the mood enhancing effect is not really because of anything in the chocolate, but because of the good taste. They declared the effect to be due to "emotional eating".[9]

The "emotional eating" effect has been challenged by a more recent double-bind study. This study compared three drinks that all tasted exactly the same: so, they controlled for taste. The first dark chocolate drink contained 500mg of cocoa polyphenols, the second contained only 250mg and the third had none. The study included seventy-one people and lasted for thirty days. Once again, the study demonstrated that chocolate significantly effects mood. But this well controlled study found that the high dose polyphenol chocolate improved calmness and contentedness significantly better than the low dose and the no dose chocolate.[10] So, while the tie breaking match has yet to declare a final victory between the dueling studies, it can be said that eating dark chocolate—for whatever reason—improves mood, and that it seems to be because of the polyphenols in the dark chocolate.

Chocolate can also elevate your mood and energize your mind after a hard mental workout. A double-blind, placebo-controlled study of healthy students found that their cognition and mood were significantly better after "highly effortful cognitive processing" when they drank cocoa beverages containing 520mg and 994mg of flavanols than when they drank a placebo cocoa drink with only 46mg of flavanols. So, the chocolate made them think better and feel better. The 520mg dose also significantly improved their mental fatigue. An odd feature of this study is that the 520mg dose seemed to work better than the 994mg dose.[11]

So, can treating yourself to some rich dark chocolate help when your mood is more in need of therapy? Can it help even when you are suffering from stress and anxiety? The early indicators are that it can.

Aside from suffering from some degree of anxiety, the people included in this study were healthy. They were between eighteen and thirty-five in age, and, while some of them only had low-anxiety, some of them were suffering from high-anxiety. Both groups ate 20 grams of 74% dark chocolate twice a day for two weeks. Eating dark chocolate significantly reduced urinary excretion of the stress hormone cortisol in the highly stressed people. Several other metabolic markers of anxiety also descended in a trend toward the levels in the low-anxiety group. The researchers concluded that this study provides "strong evidence" that dark chocolate reduces stress hormones and normalizes what they called "metabolic signatures of stress".[12]

A second study has found that chocolate can do for stress what the last study found it could do for anxiety. The study included sixty-five healthy men, and it was placebo-controlled. The men got a single 50 gram serving of 72% dark chocolate (containing 125mg of epicatechin). They were then exposed to a stressful situation. The men who got the chocolate had significantly lower levels of the stress hormones cortisol and adrenaline than did the men who got the placebo. This study suggests that the way chocolate is working is by protecting the body from stress at the level of the adrenal gland, which is the body's command central in the fight against stress.[13]

Dark chocolate may also protect you from some of the ill effects of stress on your health. When healthy men ate either 50g of flavanol-rich dark chocolate or a flavanol-free placebo bar and then underwent a social stress test, the chocolate bar prevented stress induced inflammation. The researchers say that this action could help prevent the negative effects of stress on heart health.[14]

It has long been believed that chocolate can make you feel more content. Now the science is suggesting that it really can. And the science is coming with the extra surprise that eating chocolate can make your brain not only calmer, but smarter.

PART 5:

Chocolate and Weight

CHAPTER 10

Chocolate and Weight: The Biggest Misconception

Okay. So now the question you've been asking since the beginning of the book. We probably should have just put this chapter first, because, up to now, you've probably been accepting everything we've said with reservations. You've probably been wishing it were all true while still being skeptical. Because, after all, even if chocolate is good for your heart and your blood sugar and your brain, you still can't really eat it because it's fattening. Right?

Even the researchers of several of the studies we've cited couldn't hold back that reservation. Several of them, while reporting their unexpectedly positive findings couldn't resist adding in their conclusion the caution to be moderate because, after all, chocolate is fattening. The caution wasn't based on their data. It was just common sense: everyone knows that chocolate is fattening.

But how do we know that?

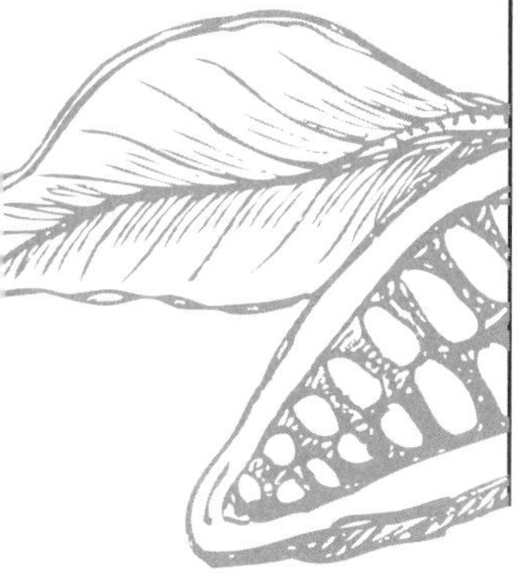

So, here comes the best news in the book. At least six studies have looked at the question of chocolate and body fat. And the good news is that not one of them has found that dark chocolate is fattening. And the news gets even better than that.

Chocolate Doesn't Affect Weight Gain

The early studies assuaged people's fears with the surprising discovery that eating dark chocolate did not affect weight. The studies were counterintuitive but clear. The first looked at overweight people who were put on an exercise program. It found, to no one's surprise at the time, that, although dark chocolate did improve their health in many ways that we have already seen, it did not improve the effects of exercise on body fat. But it didn't hurt either: it had no effect.[1] Score one for the chocolate eaters.

The second study looked at the effect of dark chocolate on type 2 diabetics. And again, it found that chocolate benefitted them—it significantly increased HDL cholesterol—without being fattening. The dark chocolate had no effect at all on weight.[2]

And Now, the Best News of All

But then the news got better still. Just as it was unbelievable but true that dark chocolate improves blood sugar, it turned out that dark chocolate not only didn't make you gain weight, it helped you lose it!

The first hint came in 2012 when a letter was published in the journal ***Archives of Internal Medicine***, a publication of the American Medical Association. It was just a hint, because it was a preliminary study and because it was published as a letter, not as a peer reviewed article. But it was an exciting hint. The researchers looked at the body mass index (BMI) of 1,018 healthy adults. BMI is a measure of weight relative to height. Their shocking discovery was that people who eat chocolate more frequently have lower BMIs than people who eat chocolate less frequently or not at all (it was also shocking to us to discover that there were people who ate chocolate not at all!). Strangely, the study found that it was not the amount of chocolate eaten that was associated with lower BMI but the frequency with which it was eaten. People who eat chocolate more often are thinner.[3]

How would this preliminary hint hold up under closer scrutiny? It may sound too good to be true, but when researchers looked at 1,458 adolescents between the ages of 12.5 and 17.5 years, they found that eating more chocolate is associated with lower levels of total and central fatness, body fat and waist circumference. Read that again if you need to, but it will say the same thing: eating more chocolate gives you less fat and makes you thinner.[4]

Another study has found the same thing. Normal weight obese syndrome (NWO) refers to a condition in which there is excessive body fat even though there is normal BMI. The condition is associated with a higher risk of cardiovascular disease. As you now know, dark chocolate is good for preventing cardiovascular disease. So, researchers tried giving fifteen women with NWO 100 grams of 70% dark chocolate every day for a week. It should no longer come as a surprise that the dark chocolate quickly helped them to improve their HDL cholesterol and the ratio of LDL and total cholesterol to HDL cholesterol. But the real surprise of the study was that eating dark chocolate reduced abdominal circumference.[5]

Yet another study looked at men and women and asked some of them to follow a low-carb diet with 1.5 ounces of 81% dark chocolate, some of them to follow the same low-carb diet without the chocolate and some of them to eat whatever they want. And the good news is, the group who ate the chocolate had significantly more weight loss. After only three weeks they had lost 10% more weight. As the study went on, the low-carb group began to put the weight back on, while the chocolate group continued to lose weight.[6]

These studies may be even more important than they seem at first. They not only show that treating yourself to dark chocolate helps you to lose weight, they show that it helps you to lose abdominal fat. And losing abdominal fat may be the most important kind of weight loss for living a longer life. They also suggest that dark chocolate can prevent the rebounding yo-yo effect of dieting.

So, now you can start getting excited about the news in this book. Against common knowledge and common sense and against the constant cautions even by research scientists, dark chocolate is not fattening: it's a weight loss food!

PART 6:

The Many Other Benefits of Chocolate

CHAPTER 11

The Antioxidant Power of Chocolate

As you have seen in many of the studies in the earlier chapters of this book, the antioxidant flavonoids make a significant contribution to dark chocolate's status as a super food. Dark chocolate is a very rich source of a powerful group of flavonoids known as polyphenols. The polyphenols found in chocolate are known as flavanols, or≠ and include catechin, epicatechin and proanthocyanidins. Dark chocolate also includes the flavonoid-like resveratrol.

Flavonoids are found in many of the most significant health promoting foods and herbs. Recent research has revealed, though, that the overall antioxidant power of dark chocolate is greater than that of "many antioxidant vegetable extracts purported to increase the body's oxidative defense."[1]

Remember, though, to get the antioxidant benefit of chocolate, the chocolate has to be rich in polyphenols, and that means that it has to be dark chocolate, cocoa powder or baking chocolate.[2]

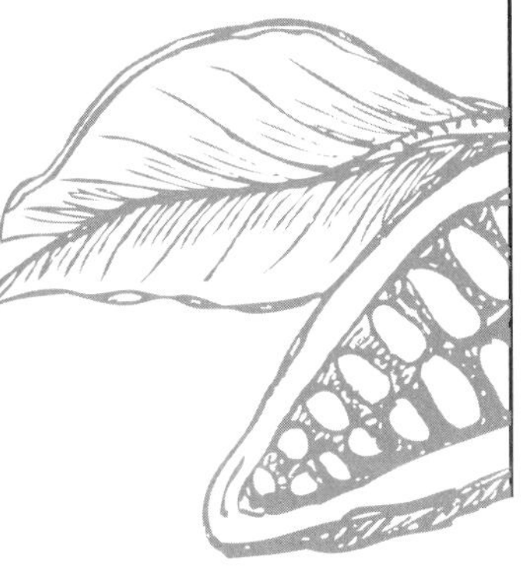

Despite all the evidence of the importance of dark chocolate polyphenols—notice that many of the studies used high polyphenol chocolate as the active intervention and low polyphenols chocolate as the placebo—not all the research has been able to show the antioxidant power of chocolate. One review of studies did not find improvements in antioxidant capacity or free radical damage. Even this review, though, did find some positive antioxidant news: the dangerous oxidation of LDL cholesterol was decreased by cocoa flavanols.[3] Several studies have found that dark chocolate protects LDL cholesterol from free radical damage, and the evidence for this important cardiovascular benefit is very strong.[4,5,6,7]

A second study that, strangely, also failed to find significant changes in total antioxidant activity also found important changes in specific antioxidant activity. As the study we just discussed found that dark chocolate protects the heart hazardous oxidation of LDL cholesterol, so this study found that dark chocolate significantly decreases oxidative damage to DNA. So, eating dark chocolate protects your cholesterol and your DNA from free radical damage. This study also found that when you eat dark chocolate—but not white chocolate—your levels of the important antioxidant epicatechin go up significantly.[8] Other studies have also shown that eating dark chocolate significantly raises your levels of epicatechin.[9] A further controlled study of healthy people found, not only that dark chocolate protects against free radical damage to LDL cholesterol, but that it does increase total antioxidant activity.[10]

Another study demonstrated the antioxidant promise of dark chocolate by looking at its effect on exercise. For two weeks before doing prolonged, exhaustive cycling, twenty men ate 40g of dark chocolate twice a day. They then ate it again two hours before cycling. A control group got a placebo chocolate. The men who ate the dark chocolate had significantly less markers of free radical damage after exercising, suggesting that dark chocolate can protect against free radical damage even in harsh conditions known to produce lots of free radicals.[11]

Other research has also shown the power of dark chocolate antioxidants in conditions known to be the harshest for free radical damage. In a study of twenty smokers, two hours after eating 40g of dark chocolate, their antioxidant status significantly increased. But there was no improvement in a group of smokers who ate the same amount of white chocolate.[12]

And one more important antioxidant study. Non-alcoholic steatohepatitis (NASH) is a kind of fatty liver disease not caused by drinking alcohol. Free radical damage plays an important role in NASH. When researchers gave people with NASH a low polyphenol placebo milk chocolate bar containing less than 35%

cocoa for two weeks, there were no important improvements. But when they gave another group the same amount of dark chocolate that was 85% cocoa and was high in polyphenols, their serum polyphenol content went up, and markers of free radical damage went significantly down, and they had significantly less liver cell death. This study shows that there are important antioxidant health benefits to eating dark chocolate.[13]

Not surprisingly then, since the flavonoids that are responsible for so many of dark chocolate's benefits are powerful antioxidants, another benefit to chalk up to eating dark chocolate is that it is an antioxidant rich super food.

Chocolate and Exercise

As we just saw, chocolate is healthy for athletes because it protects them against the free radical damage that intense exercise can create. Though that study found that chocolate can help exercisers stay healthy, it did not find any performance benefit for the athlete. Other research has found that chocolate can enhance athletic performance. People who drank chocolate milk during their recovery period after exercise were able to cycle 51% longer than people who drank a carbohydrate replacement drink and 43% longer than people who drank a fluid replacement drink. This study shows that chocolate is an effective recovery aid during workouts.[14]

More recent research has validated that positive exercise study. As we saw in chapter six on chocolate and the endothelial wall, one of the ways chocolate improves cardiovascular health is that the flavonoids in chocolate increase levels of nitric oxide. Nitric oxide also improves oxygen uptake and exercise performance. So, in a small study, nine moderately-trained men tried doing a cycling test while eating 40g a day of either dark chocolate or white chocolate. The men who ate the dark chocolate improved oxygen use and were able to cycle significantly further on a time trial than men who ate the placebo white chocolate.[15]

One of the less talked about benefits of exercise is that it strengthens not only your body, but your brain. Exercise improves cognitive function: it improves both executive function and memory. Executive function includes things like working memory, reasoning, task flexibility and problem solving. Since dark chocolate improves exercise, could it enhance the cognitive benefits of exercise?

That's exactly what researchers set out to examine in new kind of chocolate study. The study gave ten healthy, young men either a flavanol rich cocoa drink or a low flavanol cocoa drink 70 minutes before they exercised. The flavanol rich drink had 536mg of cocoa flavanols, while the placebo drink had only 38mg. The study was single-blind, meaning the men didn't know which drink they were getting, but the researchers did. 70 minutes after having the drink, the men did a moderate intensity cycling exercise for 30 minutes. They then took tests of executive function and memory.

The chocolate had no effect on memory. But it had a significant effect on executive function. In both groups, executive function improved: that's because the exercise alone improved executive function. But it improved more in the high flavanol cocoa group, meaning that eating dark chocolate before exercising enhances the beneficial effects of exercise on executive function. It is possible in this study that the chocolate improved executive function before the exercise even began.[16]

So, the evidence is mounting that dark chocolate is an emerging health food for athletes and people who exercise too.

Chocolate and Inflammation

Chocolate is loaded in flavonoids. One of the features of flavonoids we haven't explored yet is their role as one of nature's most important groups of anti-inflammatories.

Science is beginning to realize a role for inflammation in a number of conditions we don't normally think of as inflammatory, like diabetes, heart disease and Alzheimer's. So, science may discover one day that the anti-inflammatory properties of dark chocolate's flavonoids are also playing a role in its ability to fight these diseases.

The science on dark chocolate as an anti-inflammatory is still in its early stages. But test tube studies have suggested that cocoa flavanols could have anti-inflammatory ability. So, researchers decided to see what effect eating dark chocolate would have on

C-reactive protein, an important marker of inflammation.

They compared people who never ate dark chocolate to people who regularly ate dark chocolate. The ones who regularly ate dark chocolate averaged 5.7g a day. What they discovered is that the ones who regularly enjoyed dark chocolate had lower levels of C-reactive protein, meaning that eating small amounts of dark chocolate could fight inflammation. The amount of dark chocolate that was beneficial was 5.7-6.7g a day: amounts above that may no longer be anti-inflammatory.[17]

This study found that small amounts of dark chocolate have anti-inflammatory powers but that at higher amounts—over 6.7g a day—this super food loses its powers. A different study, though, that looked at different markers of inflammation, found even better results. This controlled study found that a 40g serving of cocoa powder had significant anti-inflammatory powers.[18]

Other studies have also found significantly decreased levels of C-reactive protein with daily intake of high flavanol chocolate,[19] and a meta-analysis of placebo-controlled studies concluded that dark chocolate flavanols significantly decrease C-reactive protein.[20] And, as we saw in the section on mood in chapter eight, dark chocolate possesses other important anti-inflammatory benefits.[21]

So being an anti-inflammatory food may turn out to be yet another beneficial property of dark chocolate.

Chocolate and Pregnancy

Food cravings when you're pregnant? Treat yourself to a box of chocolates! Chocolate, it turns out, is good for you when you're pregnant too.

Preeclempsia is a common and potentially serious complication of pregnancy. Blood pressure goes up, there is fluid retention and protein is lost through the urine.

Several natural nutrients have been shown to help, including calcium, magnesium, vitamin C, vitamin E, dandelion leaf, hawthorn, nettle and . . . chocolate!

Two studies have found a tremendous benefit to eating chocolate. The first found that a marker of chocolate consumption (theobromine in umbilical cord serum) was associated with a 69% decreased risk of preeclempsia. It found that women who ate chocolate at least five times a week during the first trimester were 19% less likely to develop preeclempsia; eating chocolate at least five times a week in the last trimester reduced the risk by an even better 40%.[22]

The other study found that eating only one to three servings of chocolate a week in the first trimester reduced the risk of preeclempsia by 43%. Eating more was even better: four or more servings a week bumped the protection up to 48%. Third trimester chocolate eating was associated with a 44% reduced risk. The researchers concluded that eating chocolate is associated with a significant reduction in the risk of preeclempsia.[23]

And preventing preeclempsia is not the only reason to enjoy a dark chocolate bar or two. An intriguing study looked at the overall effects of eating dark chocolate while pregnant. The study included ninety pregnant women. And, here's the good news. Half the women were told just to continue eating chocolate the way they always have. The other half were told to eat a 30g bar of 70% dark chocolate every day. The women who ate the dark chocolate daily had significantly lower systolic and diastolic blood pressure and significantly lower liver enzymes. The dark chocolate also seemed to positively affect their blood sugar, and it had no effect on weight. The researchers actually concluded at the end of the study that "A moderate amount of high-cocoa-content chocolate could be a valuable supplemental food in pregnancy".[24] So, next time someone chastises you for eating a chocolate bar while pregnant, you can tell them that it's a valuable supplement, like a maternal multivitamin!

Chocolate and Intestinal Health

It tastes way better than yoghurt! And now research suggests that dark chocolate can positively affect the balance of good and bad bacteria in your intestine.

This four week study gave either a high flavanol chocolate or a low flavanol chocolate to twenty-two healthy people every day. The high flavanol chocolate had 494mg of cocoa flavanols and the low flavanol one acted as a placebo with only 23mg of flavanols. The people who got the real chocolate had significantly increased numbers of the healthy bifidobacteria and lactobacilli bacteria. These are the type of bacteria that are beneficially supplemented as probiotics. The real chocolate also led to significantly decreased numbers of an unhealthy strain of bacteria that is associated with diseases like inflammatory bowel disease and colon cancer.

This is the first study to show that chocolate positively affects the balance of good and bad bacteria in the intestine.[25] Other studies have also found that eating chocolate has gastrointestinal benefits.[26] One study has suggested that supplementing cocoa husks, which are rich in fiber, may help children who are suffering from constipation.[27]

Chocolate and Chronic Fatigue Immune Dysfunction Syndrome

Chronic Fatigue Syndrome (CFS), now called Chronic Fatigue Immune Dysfunction Syndrome (CFIDS), is a life debilitating and difficult to treat condition. Because so little is known about how to treat it, a study showing important benefits of chocolate is particularly exciting.

In this small, double-blind study, ten people with CFIDS and severe fatigue were given either a 15g 85% dark chocolate bar or a placebo chocolate bar three times a day. Over the eight weeks of the study, fatigue continued to get worse in the placebo group but improved significantly in the dark chocolate group. The ability to work, according to a Residual Functional Capacity assessment, continued to deteriorate in the placebo group but improved significantly in the dark chocolate group. The Residual Functional Capacity assessment is a test used to determine if a person is eligible for disability or if he can still work. This real world study suggests the exciting possibility that simply eating dark chocolate regularly can significantly improve life for people who are crippled by CFIDS.[28]

Chocolate and Sunburn

Dark chocolate with your watermelon? It turns out that chocolate is the perfect summer food because chocolate protects against sunburns.

Twenty-four women were told to drink either a high flavanol cocoa beverage containing 329mg of flavanols or a low flavanol placebo chocolate beverage containing only 27mg of flavanols. The high flavanol drink is the equivalent of eating a 100g dark chocolate bar each day. The study lasted twelve weeks.

Skin sensitivity to UV irradiation was significantly lower in the high flavanol chocolate group; whereas, there was no improvement in the placebo chocolate group. Skin density and thickness, skin roughness and scaling and skin hydration all improved significantly in the dark chocolate group but not in the placebo group.

The researchers concluded that regularly consuming dark chocolate offers substantial protection against UV light and maintains skin health.[29] Other research has also found that high flavanol dark chocolate protects your skin from the harmful effects of the sun's UV rays.[30]

And chocolate not only protects your skin from the sun's damage, it can even help reverse the damage that has already been caused by the sun. Sixty-two women between the ages of forty-three and eighty-six who had wrinkles on their faces caused by sun exposure—known as photo-aging—took part in a twenty-four week long double-blind study. One group drank a placebo drink, while the other drank a high-flavanol cocoa drink containing 320mg of flavanols each day. Skin roughness improved significantly more in the cocoa group: an 8.7% improvement versus only 1.3% in the placebo group. Skin elasticity also improved significantly more in the chocolate group.[31]

Chocolate and Your Teeth

Here's another counterintuitive one: we already saw that chocolate is good for your weight, and now it turns out that it's good for your teeth too. Well, maybe.

The study wasn't on eating chocolate but on using a mouth rinse that contained cocoa bean husk extract. When the rinse was compared to a placebo rinse, it did a way better job of reducing a type of bacteria, known as ***Streptococcus mutans***, that is strongly linked to cavities. Compared to the placebo rinse, there was a 20.9% decrease in ***Streptococcus mutans*** and a 49.6% reduction in plaque.[32]

Chocolate and Your Eyes

It helps every other part of your body, so why shouldn't chocolate be good for your eyes, too? Just when we thought we were finished this book, a new study came out suggesting, for the first time, that eating dark chocolate might also be beneficial for vision.

This novel randomized, single-blind study gave thirty people who had no eye disease either a dark chocolate bar or a milk chocolate bar and then tested their eyes about two hours later. The people who got the dark chocolate bar had significant improvement in small-letter contrast sensitivity as well as slight improvements in large-letter contrast sensitivity and visual acuity compared to the milk chocolate group. When all the test scores were combined, compared to eating milk chocolate, there was significant improvement after eating dark chocolate.

These are important real world measures of vision because visual acuity tells you how big something has to be before you are capable of seeing it, and contrast sensitivity tells you how much something has to contrast with its background before you can see it.

This study suggests then that, at least as a short term effect, dark chocolate can improve your ability to see. Future research will have to see how long this beneficial effect actually lasts and what effect regularly eating dark chocolate would have.[33] And, this study seems not to be an isolated fluke. You might remember from Chapter 9 on Chocolate and Cognition that one study found that people who ate dark chocolate performed significantly better on tests of contrast sensitivity (a full 13.3% better) and visual motion detection.[34]

PART 7:

Creative Cooking with Chocolate

Onto the Fun Part!

We have discovered why you should eat more dark chocolate; now you get to eat it!

When you think of chocolate, you think of snacks and desserts. But, these recipes are really intriguing because in addition to desserts, most of them show you how to get dark chocolate into starters, salads, soups and main courses.

Here's a whole bunch of ways to get healthy, delicious dark chocolate into your diet.

Notes

- Whenever a recipe calls for milk, vegans can substitute soy, rice or almond milk
- Whenever a recipe calls for cheese, vegans can substitute their favourite vegan cheese
- A note on sweeteners: We have tried to give healthier versions of the desserts as an option. All the desserts are healthier than traditional versions because of the presence of dark chocolate instead of milk chocolate.

  If you want the more traditional taste and texture, you can use the sugar called for in the ingredients; if you want a healthier and still delicious version, you can substitute the stevia or dark

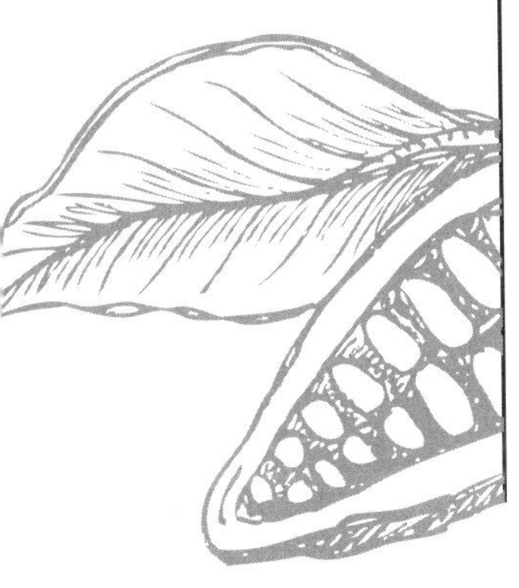

maple syrup option. Even the sugar option is healthier than the traditional versions because we have used dark cane sugar instead of white or brown sugar. Cane sugar still has all the fiber and minerals that are removed from refined sugar.

Stevia is a healthy herb that is very sweet. Beware that, if you are substituting stevia or maple syrup, you may have to adjust the amount of liquid you are using.

- A note on fats: Sometimes, there is a choice between butter and non-hydrogenated margarine.

  The story of what makes a fat a good fat or a bad fat is really the story of hydrogen. Fats contain long strings of carbon molecules. If every one of those carbon molecules is bound to as many hydrogen molecules as it can carry, then it has been filled, or saturated, with hydrogen. This is a saturated fat. If one or more carbon molecules are not saturated with hydrogen, that fat is unsaturated fat. If one carbon molecule is unsaturated, the fat is a monounsaturated fat (from the Greek *mono*, meaning one); if more than one carbon molecule is unsaturated, the fat is a polyunsaturated fat (from the Greek *poly*, meaning many).

  Saturated fats are solid at room temperature and come primarily from animal foods like meat and dairy, and they are bad for you. Unsaturated fats, which come mostly from plant foods, are good for you.

  So, which should you use, butter or non-hydrogenated margarine? Use butter if you want a natural product or if you enjoy the taste. But, if you do use it, remember two things. Butter is a saturated fat, so it is not as healthy for you. And, as you remember from the earlier chapters, some studies do show that milk neutralizes the beneficial effects of dark chocolate. Butter is made from milk. So butter might neutralize the health benefits of putting dark chocolate in your recipes. What about margarine? Hydrogenated oil is found in some packaged foods. It is also found in many margarines. Now that you know the difference between the bad saturated fats and the good unsaturated fats is the hydrogen, you can easily see why fats saturated with hydrogen (hydrogenation) are bad for you. Hydrogenated fat is exactly what it sounds like. They take unsaturated vegetable fat and add hydrogen to it: they hydrogenate it. In other words, they take a healthy, unsaturated vegetable oil and make it into an unhealthy saturated fat. That's why many margarines are bad for you.

Notice that in our recipes, we have recommended non-hydrogenated margarine. That means that the vegetable oils have not had hydrogens added and are still unsaturated fats. That is, they are healthier for you. That's is why we use them in the recipes and recommend them. ***Non-hydrogenated*** margarines are now very easy to find.

Some recipes also call for first cold pressed extra virgin olive oil. Olive oil is a monounsaturated fat and is really good for you. It is a good oil to use raw or when cooking. Flaxseed oil is a polyunsaturated fat: it is extremely healthy and a great oil to use raw.

- Always use dark cocoa powder when recipes call for cocoa powder, unless it says otherwise: it is simply healthier.
- Cocoa raw (powder) or cocoa nib means tiny little raw cocoa pieces, dark: it will usually say they are tiny little nibs in the recipe.
- For chocolate chips, unless it says otherwise, always use dark.

RECIPES

STARTERS

Lentil Walnut Spread

The lentils pair very well with the walnuts, spices and the dark cocoa nibs in this one. Serve with crackers or crunchy bread.

¾ cup dry green lentils
¼ cup walnuts, pieces
2 - 3 scallions, chopped small
2 Tbsp cocoa nibs
salt and pepper to taste
¼ tsp cumin seeds
¼ tsp cinnamon powder
pinch of chili powder
2 ½ - 3 cups strong vegetable stock

Place the lentils, 2 ½ cups of the stock and the cocoa nibs in a pot.

Turn to high heat and bring to a boil, stirring now and then, then turn to medium low heat, partially cover, and cook for about 45 minutes, or until the lentils are soft. Stir as needed, and add more liquid as needed.

If there is extra liquid left over, keep about 1 Tbsp worth, and drain the rest, to use elsewhere. Place the cooked lentils, walnuts, scallions, salt and pepper, cumin, cinnamon and chili powder in a bowl and mix well, adding the 1 Tbsp of stock if needed.

Serve hot or at room temperature.

Guacamole with Chocolate Nibs

Inspired by the guacamole I discovered in Guatemala, this is a twist on an old favourite.

1 large ripe avocado, skinned, pitted and mashed
the juice of ½ of a lime
1 - 2 crushed dried chili peppers: depends on how hot you like it
2 finely chopped green onions
1 very large garlic clove, peeled and minced
1 tsp raw cocoa, more like tiny crushed nibs
freshly chopped cilantro, about 1 tsp

Mix everything together, except the cilantro, and place in a bowl.

Decorate with the cilantro.

Serve with nachos or crackers or whatever you like.

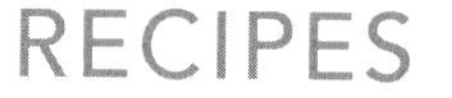

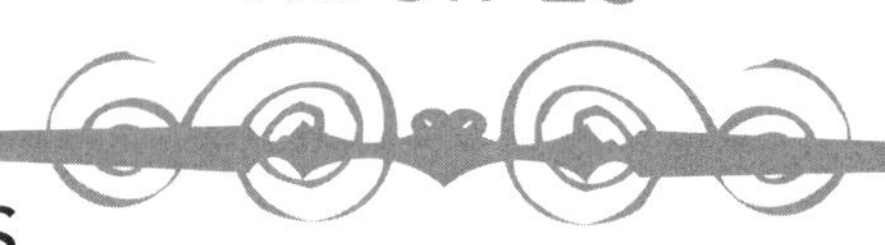

STARTERS

Sweet & Nutty Chocolate Spread

A great appetizer that feels a bit naughty: chocolate for an appetizer, not just dessert.

12 honey dates, pitted
2 Tbsp and 1 tsp of cocoa powder, dark
¼ cup sunflower seeds
6 cashews
¼ cup peanuts
1 Tbsp of dark maple syrup, to bind
1 tsp, or more, water for texture.

Place everything in a food processor and blend until smoothish. Serve with whole grain crackers.

Fig & Chocolate Spread

Simple to make and delicious.

6 fresh figs
2 Tbsp and 1 tsp of dark cocoa powder
2 Tbsp dark maple syrup
8 walnut halves
4 cashews
up to 1 tsp of water, more if needed, for texture

Place everything in a food processor and blend until smoothish.

Serve with small crackers.

RECIPES

STARTERS

Stuffed Mushrooms with a Hint of Cocoa

A great twist on a classic. The flavours go so well together, it may become the new favourite.

12 button mushrooms: remove the caps and keep, and slice thinly and into small pieces

1 Tbsp olive oil

1 very small white onion, chopped finely

1 Tbsp cocoa pieces

2 Tbsp crushed peanuts

1 tsp red pepper flake: more if you like it hotter

salt and pepper to taste

½ cup strong veggie broth mixed with 1 Tbsp of peanut butter.

In a frying pan, on medium heat, place the oil and the onion and sauté for about 5 minutes.

Add the thinly sliced, chopped, mushrooms and sauté for a few minutes.

Add the cocoa pieces, peanuts, red pepper flakes and a good grinding of black pepper and some salt, to taste, add 1 Tbsp of water and cook for a couple of minutes.

Stuff the mixture into the mushrooms, and place them in a cooking dish, stuffing side up, and pour the extra stuffing over them, and then pour the broth over them, and bake for about 30-40 minutes at 375F.

Cover for the first 15 minutes. Mushrooms should be cooked.

Don't worry if some of the stuffing falls out, it is fine, just eat with a fork.

SALADS

Avocado Salad with Chocolate

An easy, delicious starter.

3 avocados, peeled and pitted and sliced
1 cup orange juice
1 tsp raspberry vinegar or balsamic vinegar
3 oz of dark chocolate
2 tsp shredded coconut
1 Tbsp dark maple syrup

Place the avocado slices on plates.

Meanwhile, place everything else in a pot, on medium low heat, and cook, stirring and melting the chocolate.

Heat 3-5 minutes, stirring.

Then serve, poured over the avocado slices.

SALADS

Black Bean, Corn and Avocado Salad

A great combination of flavours.

19 oz cooked black beans, you can use canned, drained and rinsed

1 cup cooked corn

1 large avocado, pitted, peeled and sliced thinly

2 scallions, chopped

1 large tomato, chopped

1 tsp cilantro, chopped fine

2 Tbsp first cold pressed extra virgin olive oil

1 Tbsp lime juice, or one lime, the juice of

1 tsp lime zest, chopped tiny

¼ tsp cayenne pepper, more if you like it hotter

1 Tbsp cocoa nibs

Salt and pepper to taste

In a large bowl, place the beans, corn, avocado, tomato, scallions and cilantro.

Mix together the olive oil, lime juice and zest, cayenne pepper, cocoa nibs, and salt and pepper.

Pour over the salad.

RECIPES

SOUPS

Coconut Spiced Red Lentil Soup

A really well flavoured soup that I first had a version of at a friend's house.

1 Tbsp first cold pressed extra virgin olive oil

1 large onion, peeled and chopped

3 garlic cloves, peeled and minced

1 large carrot, diced

½ of a red pepper, cut up small

1 inch ginger, peeled and minced

½ cup dried yellow split peas

1 ½ cups dried red lentils

10 cups strong veggie stock, more, if needed

½ tsp fennel seed

1 ¼ tsp cumin powder

¾ tsp coriander powder

¼ tsp cinnamon powder

salt to taste

lots of black pepper, to taste

¼ tsp red pepper flakes, or more, to taste

¼ tsp turmeric powder

pinch of cloves

1 Tbsp cocoa nibs

¾ can of coconut milk

1 lime the juice

1 tsp lime zest

In a soup pot, place the onion and the oil and sauté on medium low heat for about 5 minutes.

Add the garlic, ginger, carrot and red pepper. Stir around for 2 minutes.

Add the spices, cocoa nibs and stir for 1 minute.

Add the split peas and stock and cover. Bring to a boil.

Reduce to medium low heat and cook for about ½ hour. Stir now and then.

Add the lentils and cook for ½ hour. Stir now and then.

Add the coconut milk and the lime zest, heat.

Add the lime juice and serve hot.

RECIPES

SOUPS

Spiced, Creamy, Avocado, Chocolate Soup

A smooth, spiced, hint of chocolate, creamy soup, that feels quite decadent.

2 large ripe avocados, remove the skins and pits

2 Tbsp dark chocolate: you can use squares, or pieces

1 ½ - 1 ¾ cups almond or soy or rice or hemp milk, more if needed, to thin a bit and blend: depends on the size of the avocados

2 Tbsp dark maple syrup

¼ - ½ tsp of chili powder, to taste

pinch of cumin powder, more if you like

Place everything in a blender and blend until smooth.

Serve right away.

RECIPES

SOUPS

Mushroom, Peanut & Spicy Red Chili Soup, with a Hint of Cocoa

A great combination of flavours that your guests will love.

1 Tbsp first cold pressed extra virgin olive oil
1 large white onion, peeled and diced
25 large button mushrooms, diced
1 - 2 tsp red pepper flakes, to taste, more if you like
3 Tbsp of crushed peanuts
2 Tbsp of peanut butter
10 cups strong veggie stock, more if needed
1 Tbsp and 1 tsp of cocoa nibs
salt and pepper to taste

In a soup pot, place the oil and the onion and sauté for about 5 minutes.

Add the mushrooms and sauté for about 3 minutes.

Add the remaining ingredients and bring to a boil.

Reduce heat to medium low, and keep covered, and cook for about 30 minutes.

Stir now and then.

Serve hot.

MAINS

Grilled Tofu with Chocolate Mole Sauce

Tofu

1 package of extra firm tofu, sliced ½ inch thick, at most.

Brown, in a frying pan, on both sides. Don't use oil. Sprinkle with chili

Mole Sauce

This sauce will adapt to lots of variations

- 1 tsp chili powder; or 1-3 green chilies, diced; or 1-2 green chilis diced and 1 habanero chili, or ancho chili, or pasilla chili, diced. You can discard seeds if you like a less fiery mole sauce, you can always use more if you like it spicier.
- 4 oz bitter sweet dark chocolate
- 1 tsp first cold pressed extra virgin olive oil
- 1 tsp balsamic vinegar
- 6 oz organic veggie soup stock
- 4 scallions, diced
- 9 or 10 cherry tomatoes, diced
- 1 large garlic clove, minced
- 1 tsp organic peanut butter
- 1 tsp lime juice
- opt. one small medium piece of diced dried mango
- pt. 1 oz tequila

Place everything in a pot, on low heat, and cook on low, stirring for about 20 minutes.

Serve over grilled tofu or anything else.

It is very good on pinto beans, black beans, tempura, grilled vegetables, corn chips, tortillas, crusty bread, fruit, crepes, wilted kale or spinach, roasted beets. It's up to you what you use it on.

If desired, you can blend it smooth. It should be thick, but liquidy.

Thin with more stock, if needed.

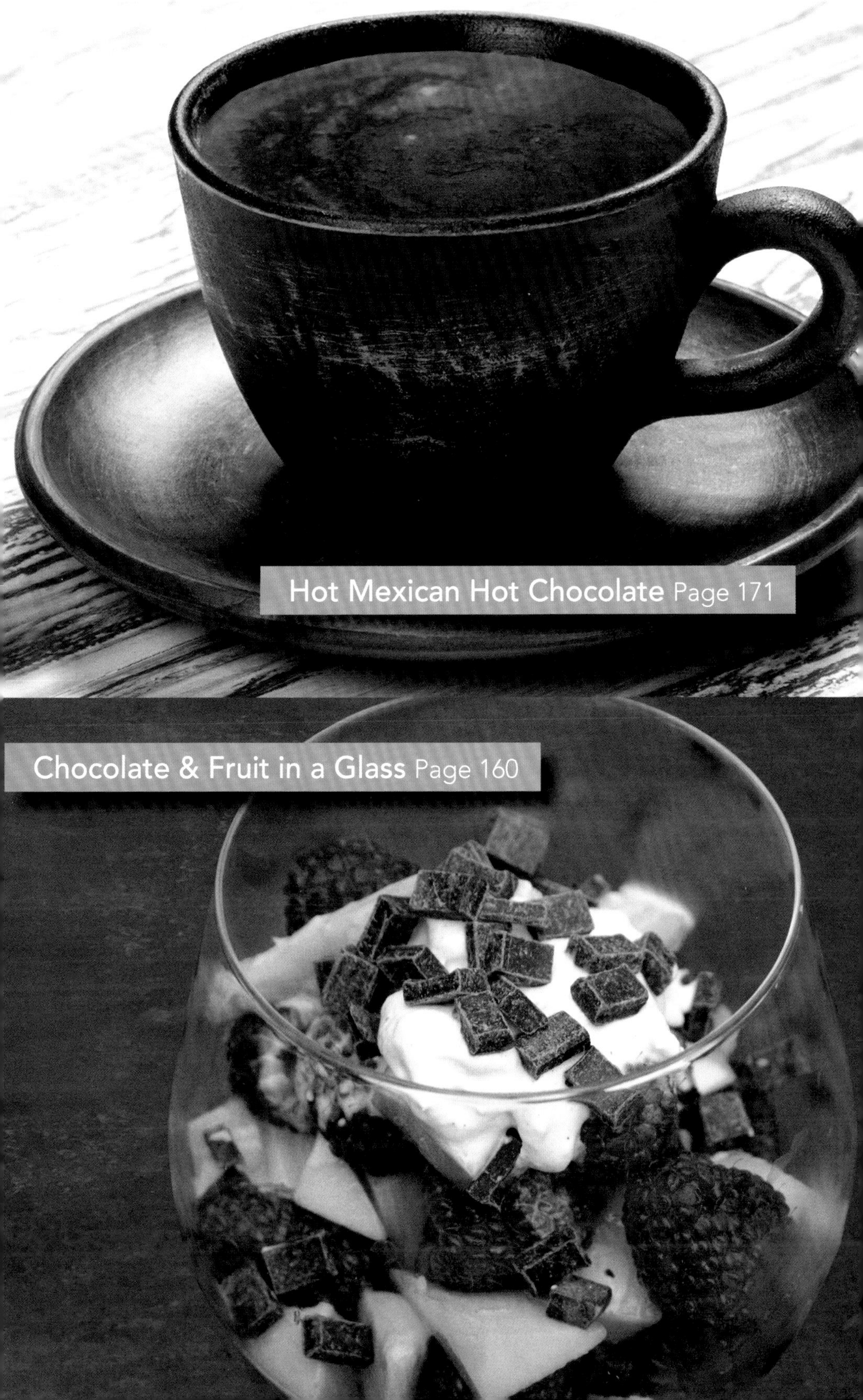

Hot Mexican Hot Chocolate Page 171

Chocolate & Fruit in a Glass Page 160

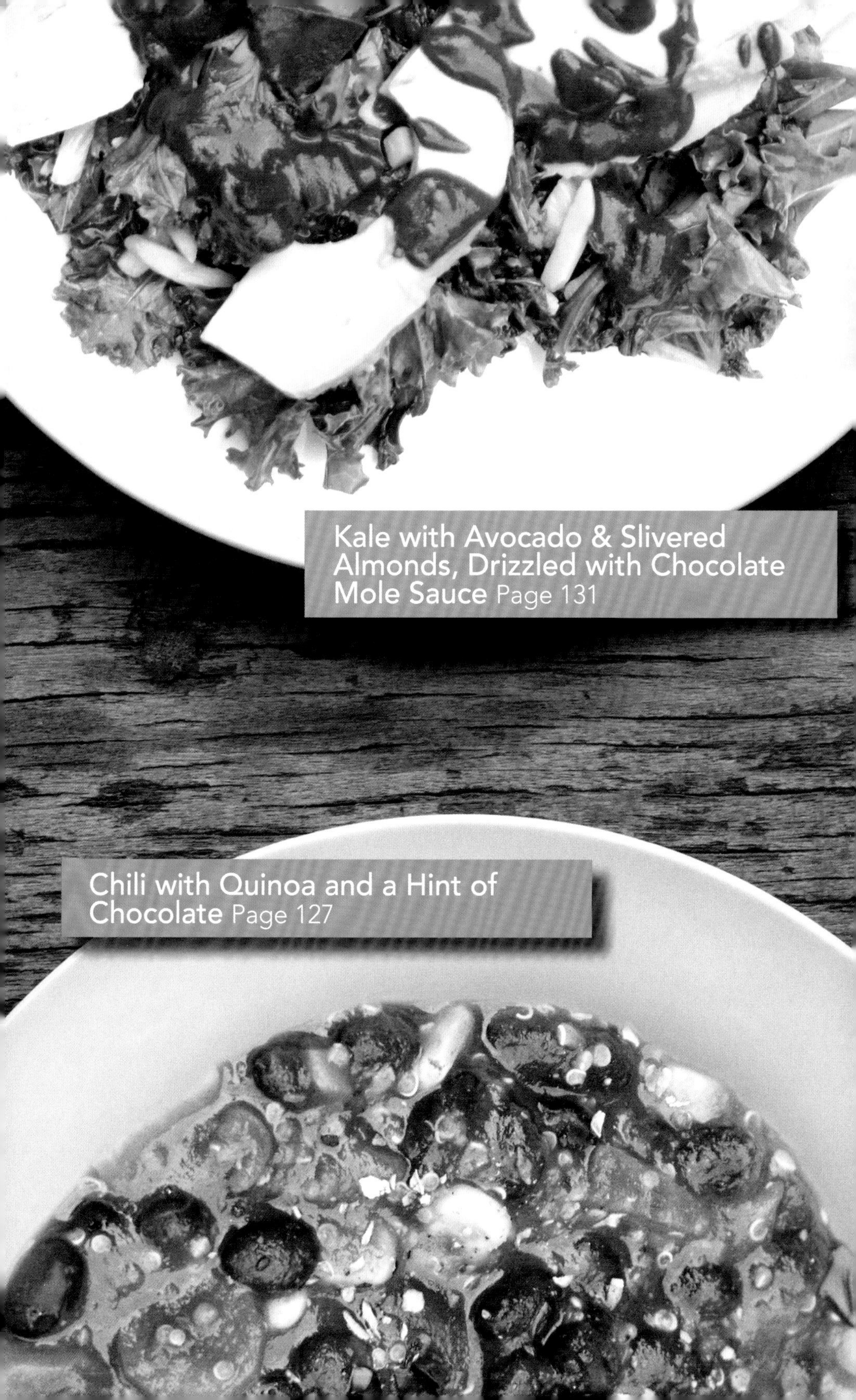

Kale with Avocado & Slivered Almonds, Drizzled with Chocolate Mole Sauce Page 131

Chili with Quinoa and a Hint of Chocolate Page 127

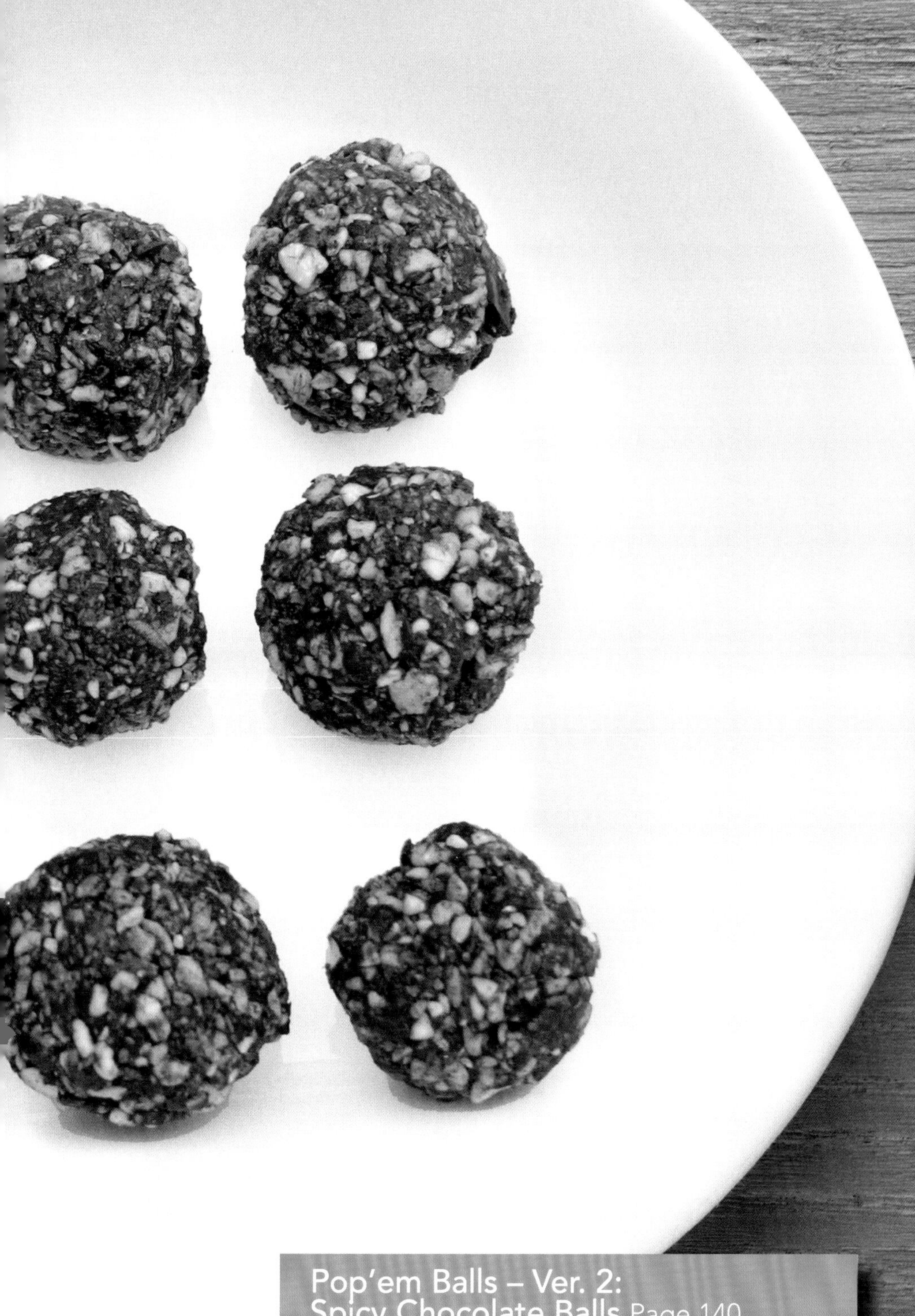

Pop'em Balls – Ver. 2:
Spicy Chocolate Balls Page 140

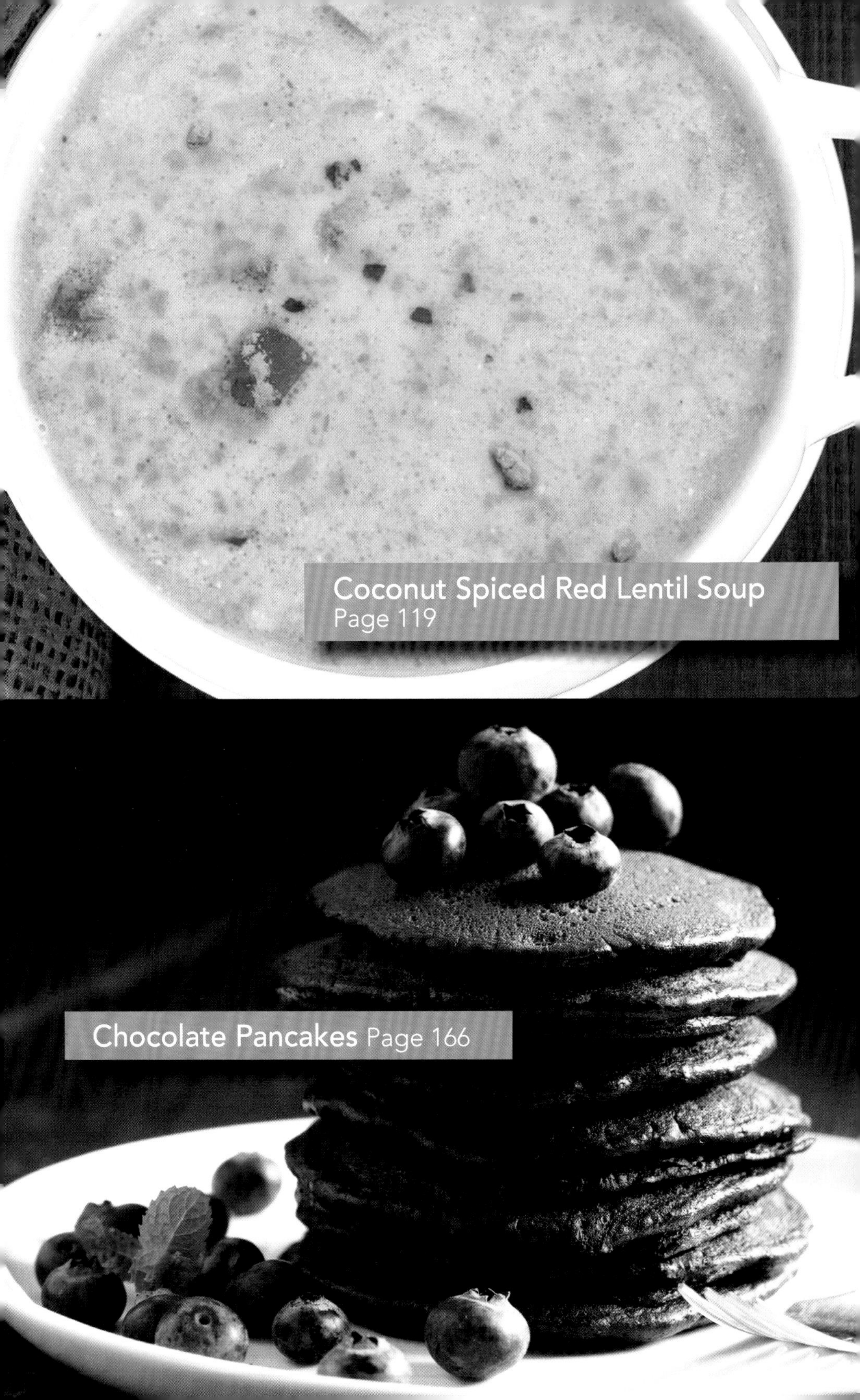

Coconut Spiced Red Lentil Soup
Page 119

Chocolate Pancakes Page 166

MAINS

Buckwheat with Cocoa Pieces, Mushrooms & Leeks

An earthy, rich tasting dish with hints of spice and cocoa.

1 Tbsp butter or non-hydrogenated margarine
1 bunch of leeks, chopped
4 large king mushrooms, chopped
12 large cremini mushrooms, sliced
10 large shiitake mushrooms, sliced
¼ tsp - ½ tsp cayenne powder, depending on how spicy you like it
1 tsp brown sesame seeds
2 Tbsp raw cocoa pieces
pinch of salt
pepper to taste: I like a good grinding
1 ¼ cup buckwheat
4 cups boiling veggie stock

In a large frying pan, place the butter (or non-hydrogenated margarine) and the leeks and cook, on medium low heat, stirring frequently, for about 5 minutes. Keep covered when not stirring. Add a bit of water as needed to prevent sticking.

Add the mushrooms and cook, stirring, for about 5 minutes. Keep covered when not stirring. Add water, as needed, to prevent sticking.

Add the cayenne powder, pepper, cocoa nibs, sesame seeds, and buckwheat and stir for about one minute.

Add the stock and cook, covered, stirring now and then, for about 1 hour, or until the buckwheat is soft.

Add salt to taste.

Serve hot.

MAINS

Grilled Tofu with Spicy Tomato Sauce with a Hint of Cocoa Nibs

A great twist.

1 block of extra firm tofu, cut in ½ inch strips
1 ½ cups tomato sauce, homemade or canned
3 very large garlic cloves, peeled and minced
1 tsp fresh lemon juice
2 dried chilies, crushed, more if you like
Pinch of cumin powder
Pinch of paprika powder
2 Tbsp raw cocoa nibs

Mix everything, but the tofu, together and brush on tofu slices.

Grill on medium heat on the barbeque, over cedar planks or mesquite wood chips, if you have them, turning now and then and brushing on both sides as they cook.

When crispy, serve.

Or, you can also make them in a frying pan. Crisp the tofu first in the frying pan, on medium heat, and then coat with the sauce and cook until crispy.

RECIPES

MAINS

Chili with Mushrooms and a Hint of Cocoa Pieces

A variation on Mexican chili that works perfectly by combining the spice of a traditional bean chili with a hint of chocolate.

- 1 Tbsp first cold pressed extra virgin olive oil
- 1 large cooking onion, peeled and diced
- 1 large garlic clove, peeled and minced
- 2 large portobello mushroom, thinly sliced, or 6 large shiitake mushrooms thinly sliced
- 3 large king mushrooms, thinly sliced
- 10 baby carrots, cut up
- 19 oz cooked black beans, you can use canned, drained and rinsed
- 28 oz diced tomatoes, you can use canned
- 2-3 tsp chili powder, depends on how hot you like it
- 1 tsp cumin powder
- ¼ tsp cinnamon powder
- ¼ tsp cayenne powder
- 1 ½ Tbsp raw cocoa pieces, tiny little nibs

In a frying pan, on medium low heat, place the olive oil and the onion and cook, stirring now and then, for about 7 minutes: keep covered when not stirring. Add a little water, if necessary, to prevent sticking.

Add the mushrooms, garlic and carrots and cook for about 15 minutes, stirring now and then. Again, keep it covered when not stirring it, and add more water, if necessary, if it sticks.

Add the remaining ingredients and cook for about 20 minutes, stirring now and then, and keeping it covered, when you are not stirring it.

Serve hot.

MAINS

Stuffed Peppers with Quinoa & Chocolate

A great high protein dish that uses the super grain quinoa, and pairs it perfectly with the antioxidant rich cocoa.

- 3 green peppers, cut in half length wise, deseed
- 2 cups cooked quinoa: cook the quinoa in a well flavoured vegetable stock, that you put one tsp of cocoa nibs in
- 3 scallions, chopped
- 2 tsp fresh dill, or dried
- ¼ tsp red pepper flakes
- ¼ tsp cumin powder
- 1 or 2 dashes of chili powder
- salt and pepper to taste
- 1 cup corn
- 2 Tbsp cocoa nibs
- 1 cup cooked black beans: you can use canned, drained and rinsed
- 3 Tbsp of salsa

Place everything, but the peppers, in a bowl and mix well.

Mound into the peppers and grill on the barbeque, closed, for about 10 minutes, on medium heat, or until cooked, or place in the oven on a baking sheet at 375°F and bake for 35-40 minutes.

MAINS

Chili with Quinoa and a Hint of Chocolate

The quinoa pairs perfectly with the cocoa pieces, the beans and corn to create a wonderful complete protein chili that is very memorable.

1 Tbsp first cold pressed extra virgin olive oil

1 cooking onion, peeled and finely chopped

½ of a red pepper, chopped

6 baby carrots, chopped small

½ cup quinoa

1 ½ cups of water

19 oz of cooked red kidney beans: you can use canned, drained and rinsed

19 oz of cooked black beans: you can use canned, drained and rinsed

1 ½ tsp - 3 tsp chilli powder, to taste

½ tsp cumin powder

¼ tsp paprika powder

¼ tsp of cayenne powder, or more, to taste

salt and pepper, to taste

opt. Red chili flakes, to taste

1 ½ Tbsp of cocoa nibs

1 tsp oregano

24 oz homemade tomato sauce, or you can use a well flavoured canned one

1 cup frozen corn

In a large frying pan, place the oil, water and the onion. On medium heat, sauté, for about 7 minutes, stirring now and then.

Add water if it sticks.

Add the carrot and the red pepper, and sauté for a few minutes, stirring now and then.

Add the quinoa and water, and cover, and cook for about 10 minutes. Stir now and then.

Add the kidney beans and black beans, the chili powder, cumin powder, paprika powder, cayenne powder, red pepper flakes, oregano, salt and pepper and cocoa nibs.

Cook for 5 minutes, covered. Stir now and then.

Add the tomato sauce, and cook for about 5 minutes, covered. Stir now and then.

Add the corn, and cook for about 5 minutes, covered. Stir now and then.

Serve hot.

RECIPES

MAINS

Cheesy Potato with Kale with a Hint of Cocoa

A delicious way of eating kale. Try all the variations: they're all good.

6 large red potatoes, skins on, thinly sliced

1 tsp of butter, non-hydrogenated margarine or first cold pressed extra virgin olive oil

pepper and salt

750 ml (3 cups) chopped fresh kale

1 Tbsp of butter or non-hydrogenated margarine

500 ml (2 cups) milk or soy milk

2 garlic cloves, minced

4 Tbsp whole wheat flour

2 eggs, beaten; or equivalent egg substitute

1 ¼ cup parmesan cheese

⅓ cup cheddar cheese, grated

1 onion, chopped

¼ tsp cayenne powder

1 Tbsp cocoa nibs

Sauté the onion in 1 tsp butter (non-hydrogenated margarine) or olive oil, until it is soft, stirring, in a frying pan, on medium low heat, add the garlic and sauté 2 minutes.

In a 9 x 13 oblong, oven proof dish, layer the potatoes, pepper, salt, kale, potatoes, onion, garlic, 1 Tbsp butter/margarine spread around, pepper and salt.

Mix together the milk, flour, eggs (or egg substitute), cocoa nibs and the cheese and lots of pepper, and pour it over the vegetables.

Cover and bake at 375°F for 45 minutes. Uncover during the last 15 minutes to brown. Eat hot.

You can substitute broccoli, spinach, cauliflower, arugula, chard, or other green vegetable for the kale.

RECIPES

MAINS

Buckwheat Crepes with Red Pepper & Onion with Hints of Cocoa

A Twist on a classic.

Wraps

310 ml (1 ¼ cups) milk
185 ml (¾ cup) buck wheat flour
2 eggs, beaten; or equivalent egg substitute
¼ tsp salt
dash of vanilla extract
2 Tbsp white flour
1 tsp cocoa powder

Place everything in a bowl and beat until very smooth.

Lightly oil a skillet and pour a very thin layer of the batter around the pan and allow it to cook on one side and then flip it over to cook the other side: about 2 minutes on each side.

Filling

1 Tbsp first cold pressed extra virgin olive oil
1 large onion, peeled and sliced
1 large red pepper, sliced
1 tsp of cocoa nibs
1-2 avocados, peeled and sliced, to taste

Sauté the onion in the oil, in a frying pan, on medium heat for about 5 minutes.

Add the red pepper and the cocoa nibs, and sauté for about 5 minutes.

Place in the crepes with sliced avocados, skins off. Roll, or fold, the crepes (really gallettes) over. Serve as is or cover with mole sauce. (See page 122 or 131 for variations).

RECIPES

MAINS

Kale with Avocados & Slivered Almonds, Drizzled with a Chocolate Mole Sauce

A great way of eating the super veggie kale: it tastes delicious in the mole sauce.

- 1 tsp first cold pressed extra virgin olive oil
- 1 large bunch of kale, cut up
- 1 large avocado, peeled and sliced thin
- ¼ cup slivered raw almonds

Place the kale in a frying pan, on medium low heat, with the olive oil and stir around until it is soft: about 5 minutes. Add a bit of water if needed.

On plates --2 of them-- mix the kale with the avocado and almonds. Serve with the mole sauce drizzled over it.

It is also good without the avocado.

Extra mole sauce will keep in the fridge to use, as needed, for a day or two.

(Chocolate) Mole Sauce

- 1- 2 green chilies, diced, to taste. Or, one green chili and one habanero chili, diced
- 4 oz bitter sweet dark chocolate
- 1 first cold pressed extra virgin olive oil
- 1 tsp balsamic vinegar
- 6 oz organic veggie soup stock
- 4 scallions, diced
- 1 medium tomato, diced, or 2 Tbsp of medium salsa
- 1 large garlic clove, minced
- 1 tsp organic almond butter
- 1 tsp lime or lemon juice
- opt. 1 tsp raw honey, if you want it sweeter

Place everything in a pot, on low heat, and cook on low, stirring frequently, for about 20 minutes. Serve over the kale mixture.

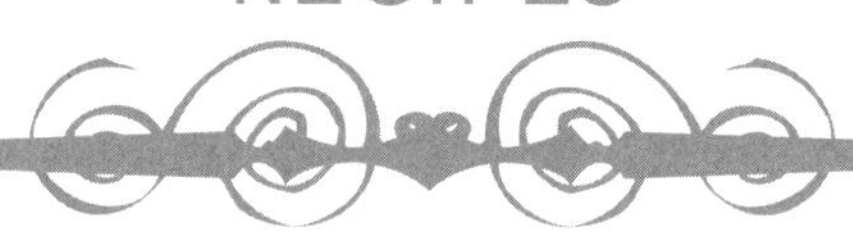

MAINS

Spicy Tofu

A spicy tofu with a hint of chocolate.

1 tsp first cold pressed extra virgin olive oil
1 pack extra firm tofu, sliced thinly
2 red chilies, dried and crushed
1 Tbsp crushed peanuts
2 Tbsp cocoa nibs
2 Tbsp peanut butter
⅓ cup strong veggie broth

Place the oil in a frying pan, on medium heat, and place the tofu in it, and brown on both sides.

Add the chilies, peanuts, nibs and cook 3 minutes.

Mix the broth with the peanut butter. Add the peanut butter and the broth. Heat and cook until the liquid is absorbed.

RECIPES

MAINS

Black Bean, Red Pepper & Avocado Burrito with a Hint of Cocoa

A great combination of flavours.

19 oz cooked black beans: you can use canned, drained and rinsed

1 small white onion, peeled and slivered

1 red pepper, cut into strips

2-3 hot peppers, diced, more if you like it hotter, to taste. Use any favorite kind, like jalapeno or red chili peppers.

½ cup tomato, diced

opt. ¾ cup cooked corn

1 large avocado, pitted and peeled and sliced thinly

opt. 1 tsp cilantro, chopped fine

¼ tsp cumin powder

1 ½ Tbsp cocoa nibs

dash of cayenne powder, to taste

½ - 1 tsp chili powder, depending on how hot you like it

salt and pepper to taste

4 whole wheat tortilla wrappers

In a frying pan, on medium heat, place the onion and cook for about 7-10 minutes in some water, until soft, stir now and then.

Add the hot peppers, red pepper and tomato, cook for about 5 minutes, stirring now and then.

And the beans, corn, cumin, cayenne powder, chili powder and cocoa nibs and cook for about 5-6 minutes, covered, stirring now and then.

Remove from the heat and mix with the avocado, cilantro, salt and pepper.

Roll in whole wheat flat breads (tortillas), like burrito wrappers, and serve hot.

RECIPES

MAINS

Mushroom Veggie Burritos

The mushrooms go very well with a hint of cocoa in this veggie burrito.

3 large king mushrooms, sliced thinly
3 large shiitake mushrooms, sliced thinly
½ of an orange pepper, cut into strips
a handful of broccoli florets
2 - 4 tsp, or more if you like it hotter, hot sauce
½ cup salsa, medium
opt. ⅓ cup cooked frozen corn
¼ tsp cumin powder
¼ tsp chili powder
¼ tsp paprika powder
one or two pinches of cayenne powder
2 Tbsp cocoa nibs
1 large avocado, peeled and sliced thinly
4 whole wheat tortilla wrappers

In a frying pan, on medium heat, place the mushrooms and cook for about 7-10 minutes in a little bit of water, stirring. Add water as needed as it cooks.

Add the orange pepper, cook for about 5 minutes, stirring now and then.

Add the broccoli, salsa, hot sauce, corn, cumin, chili, paprika, cayenne powder and cocoa nibs and cook for about 5 minutes, covered, but stir now and then.

Remove from the heat and mix with the avocado.

Roll in whole wheat flat breads (tortillas), like burrito wrappers, and serve hot.

RECIPES

MAINS

Mushroom, Avocado Quesadillas with a Hint of Cocoa

A simple, but delicious quesadilla. The mushrooms pair very well with the avocado, the chipotle peppers and the cocoa powder.

1 Tbsp first cold pressed extra virgin olive oil

2 ¼ - 2 ½ cups sliced mushrooms: shiitake, king, chanterelle, portobello, button, whatever mix you want to use

1 ½ Tbsp of raw cocoa powder, more like tiny little nibs

1 avocado, peeled and pitted

2 chipotle, or other peppers (like red chili or jalapeno): 1-2, or more: the amount and kind, depends on how hot you like it. Chipotle peppers add some smokiness to it. If you use chipotle, add ¼ tsp or so of red chili flakes when blending the avocado mixture. Red chili and jalapeno are spicy.

1 lime, the juice of

1 Tbsp olive oil

4 small whole what tortilla wrappers, or 2 large

A little olive oil for the wraps

In a frying pan, on medium-low heat, place the olive oil and the mushrooms, and sauté for about 10 to 12 minutes, add the cocoa pieces in the last few minutes.

Meanwhile, in a blender or food processor, place the avocado, peeled and pitted, the 1 Tbsp of oil, chipotle peppers (red chili flakes, if you are using them), and the lime juice. Blend until smooth.

Add to the frying pan and heat though. In another frying pan, place 1 tortilla wrap at a time in a tiny bit of olive oil.

Add some filling from the other frying pan and fold over. Cook a few minutes on both sides, until slightly browned, and serve hot. Do with all four wrappers.

RECIPES

MAINS

Thai Vegetables & Noodles with Peanut & Chocolate Flavour

A twist on a classic.

- 4 cups cooked wide whole wheat noodles, about 6oz raw: cook according to package
- 8 oz extra firm tofu, cubed
- 1 tsp of first cold pressed extra virgin olive oil
- ½ red pepper, sliced thinly
- ½ green pepper, sliced thinly
- 2 celery sticks, sliced diagonally
- 1 cup chopped nappa cabbage
- ½ cup of broccoli florets
- ½ cup cauliflower florets
- 1 cup mung bean sprouts
- 3 scallions, chopped
- 1 ½ Tbsp peanut butter
- 1 ¼ cups strong veggie broth
- 1 Tbsp cocoa nibs
- ¼ - ½ tsp, or more, cayenne powder, to taste
- salt and pepper to taste
- ¼ cup crushed peanuts
- ¼ tsp cocoa powder

Cook the pasta according to the instructions on the packet.

Meanwhile, crisp the tofu in 1 tsp of olive oil, in a frying pan, on medium heat.

Add the red and green peppers, celery and the cabbage, and cook, stirring now and then, for about 5 minutes. Add a bit of water if it sticks.

Add the broccoli, cauliflower, mung bean sprouts and scallions and cook for 3 minutes.

Meanwhile, mix the peanut butter, the hot broth, the cocoa nibs, the cayenne pepper, salt and pepper together. Add to the frying pan. Heat 2 minutes.

Mix the peanuts with the cocoa powder. Serve each serving, topped with some of the peanut, cocoa powder mixture.

RECIPES

MAINS

Quinoa, Spinach, Corn, Avocado with a Hint of Chocolate

A high protein dish you can serve hot or at room temperature.

2 cups raw quinoa

1 ½ - 2 Tbsp cocoa pieces, to taste

6 cups strong veggie broth

1 cup corn, frozen

2 avocados, pitted, peeled and sliced

1 ½ cups fresh spinach, torn up

19 oz cooked white beans or romano beans or black beans: you can use canned, drained and rinsed

salt and pepper, to taste

½ -1 tsp red pepper flakes: more if you like

¼ tsp cumin powder

1 tsp of hot sauce

¼ tsp of cayenne powder

1 lime, the juice of

Some chopped cilantro

In a large pot, place the stock and the quinoa and bring to a boil, then reduce to medium-low heat and cook for about 15 minutes, stirring now and then.

Add the cocoa nibs, and cook for 1 minute.

Add the corn, and cook for 2 minutes. Add the spinach, beans, salt and pepper, chili powder, cayenne powder, hot sauce and cumin powder and heat 2 minutes.

Add the lime juice and avocado while still on the heat.

Remove from the heat and serve on plates. Top with a little cilantro on each dish. It is also good served at room temperature.

MAINS

Veggie, Nut Burgers, with a Hint of Cocoa Nibs

A burger that goes very well with Dijon mustard on it.

1 cooking onion, peeled, roughly chopped
1 350g package of extra firm tofu
6 baby carrots,
8 raw pecans, shells removed
large handful of raw pumpkin seeds, no shells
3 raw walnuts, shells removed
¾ cup quick cook oats
pepper to taste
½ tsp paprika powder, or more to taste
1Tbsp cocoa nibs
Bragg's amino acids or soy sauce, enough to ball it up, 2-3 Tbsp: more if desired or needed
a little first cold pressed extra virgin olive oil for cooking

---

In a food processor, place everything, but the olive oil, and blend until it is smooth and begins to ball up.

Form into patties. It makes about 16.

Place each in a frying pan that has a thin coating of olive oil on it.

Cook, flipping onto both sides, on medium heat, for about 15-20 minutes. They should be golden brown on both sides.

Serve hot or cold.

You can place condiments on it, like pickles, Dijon mustard, lettuce and sprouts, or eat plain or with a hot sauce or other favorite sauce.

Pop 'em Balls

Of course, this healthy desert/snack/energy treat is a favourite from my cookbook, The All-New Vegetarian Passport, but this is a new version. And it has those healthy flaxseeds in them with essential fatty acids to prevent and treat a whole host of health problems. And they are delicious: a favourite with kids and adults alike. Take them on your next hike or keep them as a healthy snack or serve them at parties.

½ cup (125 ml) raw almonds

¼ cup (60 ml) raw sunflower seeds

¼ cup (60 ml) raw walnuts pieces, or raw pecans

1 Tbsp (15 ml) milled flaxseeds

½ cup (125 ml) unsweetened coconut, shredded

1 ¼ cups (300 ml) Thompson raisins

8 dried dates, pitted

1 Tbsp dark cocoa powder: more if you like it chocolatier

apple juice as needed, about 1 - 2 Tbsp (15 - 30 ml)

All the nuts and seeds should be without shells.

Place everything in a food processor, except the apple juice, and blend until it is fairly smooth.

Add enough juice to make it stick together, enough to form into balls: usually 1-2 Tbsp (15-30 ml) or so.

Form into small balls and allow to harden. Enjoy!

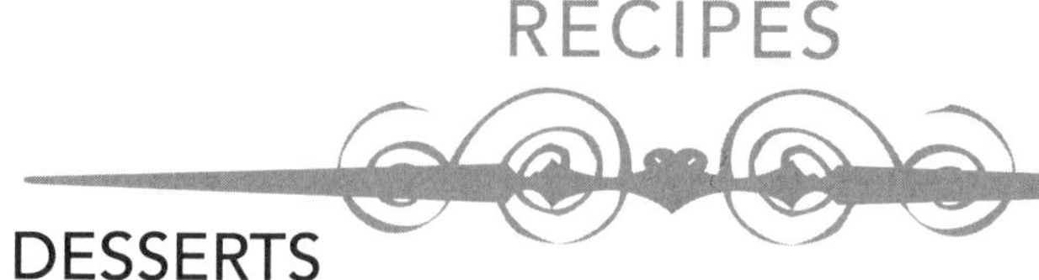

DESSERTS

Pop 'em Balls Version 2: Spicy Chocolate Balls

Spicy and good. The antioxidant rich cocoa powder and the heart healthy, spicy cayenne powder give these balls quite a health punch for a dessert.

½ cup (125 ml) raw almonds
1 cup dried dates
½ cup (125 ml) unsweetened shredded coconut
1 tsp brown sesame seeds
¼ tsp (1 ml) cayenne powder: more if you like it hotter
1 Tbsp (15 ml) pure cocoa powder
apple juice as needed

The almonds should be without shells.

Place everything in a food processor, except the apple juice, and blend until it is fairly smooth.

Add enough juice to make it stick together, enough to form into balls, usually 1 Tbsp (15 ml) or so.

Form into small balls and allow to harden. Enjoy!

Pop 'em Balls Version 3: Blueberry, Nut & Cocoa Balls

Rich in antioxidant blueberries, with their proanthocyanidines, and antioxidant rich cocoa.

¼ cup (60 ml) raw almonds
½ cup (125 ml) raw peanuts
7 - 8 cashew nuts, raw
½ cup (125 ml) dried blueberries
10 dried dates
1 Tbsp (10 ml) pure cocoa powder
½ cup (125 ml) unsweetened shredded coconut
apple juice, as needed

All the nuts should be without shells.

Place everything in a food processor, except the apple juice, and blend until it is fairly smooth.

Add enough juice to make it stick together, enough to form into balls: usually 1 Tbsp (15 ml) or so.

From into small balls and allow to harden. Enjoy!

DESSERTS

Pop'em Fruit, Chocolate & Nut Balls

More flavours of the healthy snack.

1 ¼ cups dates
½ cup raw cashews
½ cup shredded coconut
2 Tbsp chocolate chips, bitter sweet, dark, or 2 Tbsp of cocoa powder
¼ cup brown sesame seeds
2 Tbsp apple/cranberry juice

Place everything, but the juice, in the blender and blend until smooth.

Add the juice to hold it together and mix.

Form into balls and allow to harden.

Eat.

Chocolate Date Coconut Balls

An easy delicious healthy treat.

1 cup sweetened coconut
12 dried dates, pitted
2 Tbsp cocoa powder
dark maple syrup, to bind: 1 tsp - 1 Tbsp is usually needed

Place the coconut, dates and cocoa powder in a food processor and blend until smooth.

Add enough maple syrup so it will stick together but not be sticky.

Form into balls and harden in the fridge.

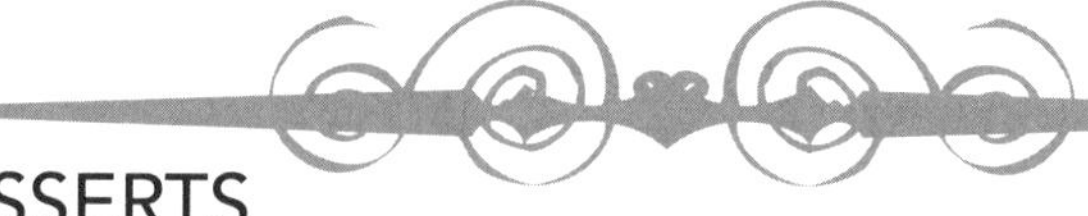

DESSERTS

Date, Fig, Chocolate & Coconut Squares

A simple, delicious treat, made with fruit and oats, so it is a healthier treat.

- ¼ cup (60 ml) butter or non-hydrogenated margarine (dairy free)
- 2 cups (500 ml) quick cooking oats
- ¾ cup (185 ml) brown cane sugar or dark maple syrup or ¾ tsp stevia
- 1 ¼ tsp (6 ml) cinnamon powder
- ¼ tsp (1 ml) salt
- ¾ cup (185 ml) shredded coconut
- 1 ½ cup (375 ml) pitted dried dates
- 4 fresh figs, chopped small
- 2 Tbsp cocoa powder
- 2 Tbsp (30 ml) fresh lemon juice
- 4 Tbsp (60 ml) apple juice

Melt the butter (or non-hydrogenated margarine) in a saucepan on low heat, stirring.

Remove from the heat.

Mix in the cinnamon, sugar or syrup or stevia, oatmeal, salt and coconut.

Mix well and press ½ of the mixture into a greased 8" x 8" (20 cm x 20 cm) baking dish.

Blend the remaining ingredients in a food processor, except the apple juice, and spread over the oatmeal mixture.

Top with the other half of the oatmeal mixture.

Pour the apple juice over top and bake at 375°F (190°C) for 30 minutes.

Apricot, Coconut Chocolate Squares

Another version of a simple delicious treat that is also made with fruit and oats, so it is a healthier treat.

¼ cup (60 ml) butter or non-hydrogenated margarine (dairy free)

2 cups (500 ml) quick cooking oats

¾ cup (185 ml) brown cane sugar or dark maple syrup or ¾ tsp stevia

1 tsp (5 ml) cinnamon powder

¼ tsp (1 ml) salt

¾ cup (185 ml) shredded coconut

1 ½ cups (375 ml) dried apricots or dried mango

1 Tbsp cocoa powder

2 Tbsp (30 ml) fresh lemon juice

4 Tbsp (60 ml) apple or cranberry juice

Melt the butter (or non-hydrogenated margarine) in a saucepan on low heat, stirring.

Remove from the heat.

Mix in the cinnamon, sugar or syrup or stevia, oatmeal, salt and coconut.

Mix well and press ½ of the mixture into a greased 8" x 8" (20 cm x 20 cm) baking dish.

Blend the remaining ingredients in a food processor, except the cranberry juice, and spread over the oatmeal mixture.

Top with the other half of the oatmeal mixture.

Pour the juice over top and bake at 375°F (190°C) for 30 minutes.

DESSERTS

Baklava with Chocolate

A Greek classic with a twist.

- phyllo pastry
- butter or non-hydrogenated margarine
- 2 ½ cups blanched almonds
- 1 ½ - 2 tsp cinnamon
- ½ cup brown cane sugar or dark maple syrup or ½ tsp stevia
- opt. 1 cup walnuts or pistachios: if you use them omit 1 cup of almonds
- 2 Tbsp cocoa powder, like tiny nibs

In a 12 x 9 oblong pan, place 4 sheets of folded phyllo pastry, brushing each one with butter (non-hydrogenated margarine).

Blend everything else together in a food processor until smooth. Add a layer of it on top of the phyllo.

Then add 4 more sheets, brushing each one with butter/margarine, another layer of filling, more brushed sheets, etc., until you have used it all up, ending with the phyllo. Sprinkle very lightly with water.

Score the top into squares and bake at 325°F for 40-60 minutes or until golden on top. Meanwhile, prepare a syrup.

Syrup

- 16 oz cane sugar or dark maple syrup
- 5 oz honey
- 6-8 oz of water
- 1 ½ tsp cinnamon
- 1 tsp cloves
- 1 tsp of cocoa powder

Bring everything to a boil, stirring all the while. Do not allow to burn.

Turn down the heat and keep at a low boil for about 15-25 minutes. Stir frequently.

Remove cloves and pour over the cooked baklava. Cut into squares. Let sit 2 hours or so before serving. Serve.

DESSERTS

Orange Chocolate Pecan Shortbread Cookies

Rich and delicious. Kind of a well-flavoured shortbread.

- 1 cup butter or non-hydrogenated margarine
- 1 cup icing sugar or dark maple syrup
- 1 tsp vanilla extract
- 1 ½ cups whole wheat flour
- 1 cup crushed pecans
- 2 Tbsp cocoa powder
- 1 orange, peeled and put through a food processor (keep 1 tsp of finely chopped rind)
- 1 tsp first cold pressed extra virgin olive oil
- 1 tsp orange extract

Cream together the butter or non-hydrogenated margarine, sugar or dark maple syrup and vanilla, then blend in the flour and cocoa powder

Add the pecans, orange, peel, orange extract and the olive oil.

Mix well.

Form into cookies and bake at 300°F for 25-30 minutes. Do not brown.

Serve.

Makes about 14 cookies.

DESSERTS

Orange, Chocolate, Bran Raisin Muffins

A chocolate hint in a fruity tasting muffin.

¾ cup bran
1 ¼ cup whole wheat flour
3 Tbsp brown cane sugar or a pinch of stevia
½ tsp salt
2 Tbsp cocoa powder
1 ½ tsp baking powder
1 orange, peeled and put through a food processor
½ cup raisins
½ cup small dark chocolate chips
1 egg or equivalent egg substitute
orange juice
2 tsp first cold pressed extra virgin olive oil

Mix everything together well.

Add orange juice if it seems a little dry.

Half fill non-stick muffin tins.

Bake at 375°F for about 15-25 minutes or until a tooth pick comes out cleanly.

Chocolate Peanut Butter Cookies

These are the best chocolate peanut butter cookies that I have ever had.

- 1 cup vegetable shortening (you may need less if you 're using stevia)
- 2 cups brown cane sugar or 2 tsp stevia
- 1 tsp vanilla
- 2 eggs, beaten; or equivalent egg substitute
- 1 tsp salt
- 5 oz tiny chocolate chips, bitter sweet dark
- 1 tsp soda in 1 Tbsp boiling water
- 1 tsp baking powder
- 2 ½ cups whole wheat flour
- 1 ¼ cups peanut butter

Mix everything together and roll into 1 ½-2 inch balls.

Press each ball down with a fork on a greased cookie sheet and bake at 350°F for 10-15 minutes or until a tooth pick comes out cleanly.

DESSERTS

Oatmeal, Almond, Coconut, Chocolate Chip Cookies

Best cookies ever.

1 ½ cups whole wheat flour

1 ½ cups brown cane sugar or 1 ½ tsp stevia

1 cup vegetable shortening
(you may need less if you're using stevia)

½ cup butter or non-hydrogenated margarine
(you may need less if you're using stevia)

1 tsp first cold pressed extra virgin olive oil

3 cups quick cook oatmeal

1 tsp cocoa powder

1 tsp cinnamon

1 tsp salt

2 cups of dark chocolate chips

1 cup shredded coconut

½ cup slivered almonds

A drop of milk/soya milk

Mix everything together well and shape into small 1 inch balls.

Place them 3 inches apart on a greased cookie sheet and press down with a fork to ¼ inch thick.

Bake at 375°F for 8-10 minutes, or until golden.

Recipe can be doubled.

Chocolate Cookies

These always do well at vegetarian food fairs, selling out very quickly.

2 cups brown cane sugar or 2 tsp stevia

½ cup soya milk
(you may need less if you're using stevia)

½ cup cocoa powder 1 tsp vanilla

½ cup butter or non-hydrogenated margarine
(you may need less if you're using stevia)

3 cups oatmeal, quick cook

1 cup shredded coconut

Boil, stirring all the while, the sugar or stevia, milk, cocoa, vanilla and butter (or non-hydrogenated margarine.)

Turn down to a low boil for 5 minutes. Do not burn.

Remove from the heat and add the remaining ingredients.

Mix well and drop off by a spoon onto a cookie sheet.

Allow to harden and serve.

DESSERTS

Chocolate Cake

Everyone has a favourite chocolate cake, and this one is mine. It uses delicious, pure dark chocolate powder and uses healthier ingredients than most cakes.

- butter or non-hydrogenated margarine for greasing the pans
- 1 ¾ cups whole wheat flour
- 2 cups brown cane sugar plus one Tbsp or 2 tsp stevia
- ¾ cup dark cocoa powder
- 1 Tbsp baking soda
- 2 tsp baking powder
- pinch of sea salt
- 2 free range eggs
- 1 ½ cups almond milk or 2% milk (you may need less liquid if you're using stevia)
- 2 Tbsp butter or non-hydrogenated margarine
- 2 Tbsp dark maple syrup
- 1 tsp vanilla extract
- dark chocolate, 2 tsp grated, for topping

Preheat the oven to 350° F. Grease, with butter (or non-hydrogenated margarine), a 12 x 9 baking pan. You can also use 2 round baking pans and make two cakes and layer them.

Sift the flour, sugar or stevia, cocoa, dark chocolate, baking soda, baking powder, and salt into the bowl together. In another bowl, combine the almond milk, butter/margarine, eggs (or egg substitute), maple syrup, and vanilla. Using an electric mixer, on low speed, slowly add the wet ingredients to the dry. Beat on high speed until smooth. Pour the batter into the prepared pan and bake for about 40 minutes, or until a toothpick or cake tester, comes out clean. Cool in the pan for 30 minutes, then turn it out onto a cooling rack and cool completely.

Ice the cake or, if using two cakes, place 1 layer, flat side up, on a flat plate or cake pedestal. With a knife, spread the top with icing. Place the second layer on top, rounded side up, and spread the icing evenly on the top and sides of the cake. Top with dark chocolate gratings.

Can also be made into cupcakes by pouring batter, ¾ full, into a cup- cake baking pan and baking, until a tooth pick come out cleanly from the cupcakes, less time than as a cake (start checking at 10-15 minutes), and then frost with icing.

Chocolate Icing

A rich, creamy icing that you can alter by adding different extracts; for example, orange or mint or nut extract can be added.

3 Tbsp butter or non-hydrogenated margarine
2 ½ cups icing sugar
A dab of soya milk
1 tsp vanilla
3 Tbsp cocoa powder for chocolate flavour

Mix together everything and whip up well.

Spread on cake or muffins and allow to harden.

Serve.

DESSERTS

Chocolate, Orange, Walnut Squares

A great desert. You can substitute hazelnuts for walnuts, if you like, for a change of taste.

- 1 orange, including the peel
- ¾ cup pitted dates
- 1 ½ cups whole wheat flour
- ½ cup butter or non-hydrogenated margarine
- ⅓ cup cocoa
- 1 cup brown cane sugar or dark maple syrup
- 1 ¼ cup walnut halves

Blend everything, except the walnuts, in a food processor until smooth.

Press into a foil lined square pan.

Cover with a layer of walnuts (about 1 ¼ cup). Press them down.

Make a sauce.

Sauce

- ½ cup brown cane sugar or dark maple syrup
- ½ cup butter or non-hydrogenated margarine
- 1 cup chocolate chips

Bring the butter (or non-hydrgenated margarine) and the sugar or syrup to a boil, stirring, and then simmer 1 minute.

Pour over the squares.

Bake at 350°F for 25-30 minutes.

Spread on a layer of chocolate chips. Bake for 2 minutes.

Allow to cool and cut into squares. Serve.

Spicy Indian Chocolate Nuts

Spicy Indian barbecue flavour in this one, with a hint of cocoa.

1 cup raw peanuts, with or without the skins
1 cup raw almonds
2 Tbsp raw cocoa: it is more like tiny nibs
½ tsp first cold pressed extra virgin olive oil, a bit more, if needed
1 tsp tandoori barbecue masala
1/8 tsp chili powder, or more
2 dashes of cayenne powder: more if you like it hotter. (I like about ¼ tsp)

Cook the nuts, in the oil, in a frying pan on medium low heat for a few minutes, stirring.

And add the other ingredients, and cook a few minutes, stirring.

Mix to coat well.

Serve.

DESSERTS

Spicy Chocolate Party Mix

These nuts are a great one for parties.

¼ cup raw sunflower seeds
½ cup raw peanuts
1 cup raw almonds
¼ cup walnuts
¼ cup raw pumpkin seeds
a handful each of pecans and cashews
1 ½ Tbsp raw cocoa powder, more like tiny nibs
½ tsp first cold pressed extra virgin olive oil
1 tsp chili powder
¼ tsp paprika powder
¼ tsp of cayenne, or more, to taste
pinch of sea salt

Heat the nuts in a frying pan until they begin to crackle.

Add the oil and the spices and mix to coat well and heat a few minutes.

Serve.

Cumin Flavoured Chocolate Seeds & Nuts

A spicy snack.

1 cup raw almonds

6 raw brazil nuts

1 cup raw pumpkin seeds

¼ cup raw sunflower seeds

1 ¼ tsp cumin seeds

¼-½ tsp chili powder, to taste,
depends on how spicy you like it: I like it spicy

1 Tbsp cocoa powder

¼ tsp cinnamon powder

pinch of sea salt

pinch of cayenne powder

1 ½-2 tsp first cold pressed extra virgin olive oil: enough
to coat the nuts without being oily

Place everything in a frying pan, on medium low heat, and cook for 2-3 minutes, stirring.

DESSERTS

Chocolate Banana Bread

I think that this is a great version of banana bread.

8 oz whole wheat flour
2 ½ tsp baking powder
2 oz butter or non-hydrogenated margarine
2 Tbsp first cold pressed extra virgin olive oil
2 oz dark cane sugar or dark maple syrup
3 oz honey
1 Tbsp dark maple syrup
3 oz chopped pecans or walnuts
1 package of dark chocolate chips, small ones
2 large bananas, without the skins and mashed
1 egg or equivalent egg substitute

Mix together the dry ingredients: flour and baking powder.

Melt the butter (or non-hydrogenated margarine) and add the honey and sugar or syrup, stir until smooth, and then remove from the heat and add the maple syrup and oil to it.

Mix into the dry ingredients.

Beat the egg (or egg substitute) and add it.

Add the bananas, chocolate chips and the walnuts and mix well.

Place in a nonstick or greased loaf tin and bake for 1 hour or so, or until a toothpick comes out cleanly.

Cut into slices and serve, hot or cold.

Pears in Chocolate Sauce

Fast and easy, this is a delicious and healthy dessert. And the pears go wonderfully well with the deep rich chocolate.

1 tsp butter or non-hydrogenated margarine

2 pears, best in the fall,
remove the cores and slice thinly, skin on

2 Tbsp cocoa powder

4 Tbsp dark maple syrup

opt. ¼ tsp of cinnamon powder

Place the butter (or non-hydrogenated margarine) in a cast iron frying pan, on medium heat, and add the pears.

Stir around for about 3-4 minutes, until the pears are soft, watch that the pears do not burn or stick.

Add the cinnamon powder and the cocoa powder and stir for 1 minute.

Add the maple syrup and stir around for about 3 minutes.

Serve hot.

DESSERTS

Chocolate & Fruit in a Glass

Pretty and delicious.

1 cup vanilla coconut yogurt

½ tsp orange extract

4 Tbsp dark chocolate chips or flakes

½ cup raspberries

1 mango, cut in pieces

Mix yogurt and extract together and place a small portion in the bottom of two glasses.

Sprinkle some dark chocolate chips or flakes and then place fruit.

Top with more yogurt mixture and sprinkle with dark chocolate

Chill for 15 minutes an serve.

Orange Chocolate Date Muffins

A great tasting muffin.

1 cup pitted dates
1 large orange, peeled
1 tsp zest of orange, chopped fine
½ cup orange juice, more if the batter seems to dry
¼ cup olive oil
2 eggs, beaten; or equivalent egg substitute
1 ½ cups whole wheat flour
¾ cup brown sugar, or sucanat
1 Tbsp baking powder
1 tsp baking soda
¼ tsp salt
2 Tbsp of cocoa powder
2-3 oz of dark chocolate chips

In a food processor, blend the dates, orange, orange, juice, zest and olive oil until smooth.

Add the remaining ingredients, except the chocolate chips, and blend well.

Pour ¾ full into greased muffin tins.

Press a few of the chocolate chips into the top of each muffin.

Bake at 375°F for 15-25 minutes, or until a tooth pick comes out cleanly.

DESSERTS

Desert Crepes

A French inspiration that is great for company or just when you want something special.

Shells

1 ¼ cup milk

¾ cup whole wheat flour

2 eggs, beaten; or equivalent egg substitute

1 tsp cocoa powder

¼ tsp salt

dash of vanilla

2 Tbsp white or whole wheat flour

Place everything in a bowl and beat until very smooth.

Lightly oil a skillet and pour a very thin layer of the batter around the pan and allow it to cook on one side and then flip it over to cook the other side: about 2 minutes on each side.

Stuff and cover with a sauce.

Filling

1 pint raspberries or blueberries

2 Tbsp raspberry jam

Heat and cook for 3 minutes.

Place some of the filling in each crepe roll.

Sauce

6 oz, semi-sweet or dark chocolate chips
1 tsp vanilla extract
1 Tbsp butter or non-hydrogenated margarine
¾ cup icing sugar
½ cup soy milk
opt. 1 Tbsp orange, Kahlua® or almond liquor
Dark chocolate shavings.

Melt together slowly, stirring on low heat until thick, smooth and bubbly. Pour a little sauce over each crepe and serve. If desire, serve with chocolate shavings.

DESSERTS

Frozen Chocolate Yogurt Dessert

A great healthy treat.

1 ½ cup plain yogurt with probiotics

2 tsp cocoa powder

one of the following, or some of each: strawberries, blackberries, raspberries, blueberries, about 2 cups, or omit fruit and use 2 Tbsp organic peanut butter

3 Tbsp soya lecithin granules

opt. 1 Tbsp maple syrup

Place everything in a blender or food processor and blend until well mixed.

Place in a covered container and freeze.

Allow to thaw in the refrigerator for a few hours and then eat.

RECIPES

DESSERTS

Chocolate French Toast

A classic, with a chocolate treat.

4 - 5 slices of challah bread or whole wheat bread if desired
2 eggs, beaten; or equivalent egg substitute
1 tsp cinnamon powder
salt to taste
dash of vanilla extract
½ cup almond or soy milk (non-dairy), more if needed
2 Tbsp cocoa powder
butter or non-hydrogenated margarine
chocolate shavings

In a large bowl, beat together the eggs (or egg substitute), cinnamon, salt, vanilla, milk and cocoa powder.

Dip the bread slices in the bowl and cover with the liquid. Place in a hot frying pan, that has been greased with butter (or non-hydrogenated margarine,) on medium heat, and cook, about 3-5 minutes, on each side, or until golden.

Spread a tab of butter or non-hydrogenated margarine on each piece. Sprinkle each slice with a bit of the chocolate shavings.

Serve hot.

DESSERTS

Chocolate Pancakes

A great breakfast that kids and adults alike love. Use dark chocolate for extra antioxidants.

- 1 cup whole wheat flour
- 1 tsp baking powder
- 2 tablespoons dark maple syrup
- ¼ teaspoon salt
- 2 tablespoons unsweetened cocoa powder
- 1 egg, or equivalent egg substitute
- 1 ½ c milk, 2%, more, if needed, to thin the batter: batter should bubble when cooking
- 2 Tbsp butter or non-hydrogenated margarine, melted
- 1 tsp vanilla extract
- 6 oz of dark chocolate chips
- opt. Some fine dark chocolate, shavings, for serving
- fresh blueberries, for serving
- dark maple syrup, for serving
- 1 tsp of butter or non-hydrogenated margarine, for frying pan

---

In a large bowl, combine dry ingredients flour, baking powder, salt, cocoa powder.

Mix together the milk, egg (egg substitute), butter or non-hydrogenated margarine), maple syrup and vanilla in another bowl.

Combine wet ingredients into the dry ingredients. Do not over mix. Add the chocolate chips.

Heat a griddle/frying pan, over medium heat, add 1 tsp of butter. Drop ¼ cup scoops of batter onto the griddle. Flip once. Cook until done, cooked through. Top each pancake with a touch of butter while still piping hot. And dust with icing sugar, if desired, and shaved chocolate, if desired. You can also add your favorite berries and/or maple syrup.

Chocolate Peanut Butter Smoothie

A great easy meal or snack

2 cups soy milk, almond, rice, or hemp milk, plain or vanilla

2 ½ Tbsp organic peanut butter

2 Tbsp cocoa powder, or more if you like

opt. 1 scoop of protein powder,
for a thicker shake: soy, rice or hemp

opt. You can also thicken with half of a peeled banana

Place everything in a blender and blend until smooth.

DESSERTS

Chocolate Almond Smoothie

A great easy meal or snack

2 cups soy milk, or rice, or almond, or hemp milk, plain or vanilla

2 ½ Tbsp organic almond butter

2 Tbsp cocoa powder, more if you like

opt. one scoop of soy, rice or hemp protein powder (for a thicker shake)

opt. ½ of a peeled banana to thicken

Place everything in a blender and blend until smooth.

Chocolate Blueberry Smoothie

A great, easy meal or snack that is loaded in antioxidants, like proanthocyanidins from the blueberries, flavonoids from the cocoa powder, and isoflavones from the soy (if you use it): a cancer fighter that is also good for your bones, heart and menopausal symptoms. It is a complete protein. And it tastes great.

1 ½ cup soy, rice, almond or hemp milk, plain or vanilla

1 cup blueberries: a little more if you like it thicker.

2 Tbsp cocoa powder, more if you like,
use dark cocoa powder for great antioxidants

Place everything in a blender and blend until smooth.

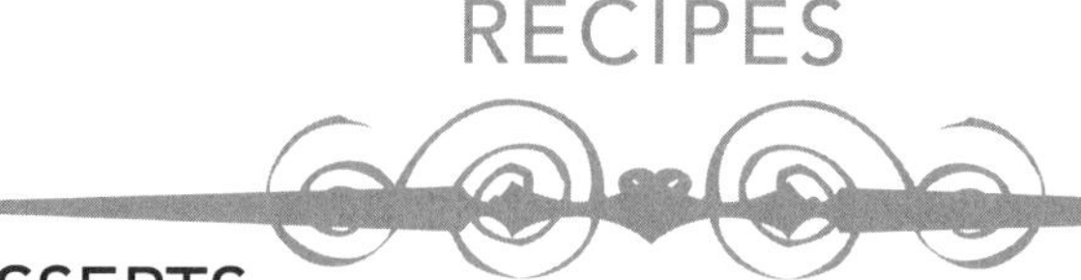

DESSERTS

Chocolate Orange Smoothie

A great pairing of chocolate and orange in a smoothie.

1 mini banana, frozen, skin off
1 cup orange juice
2 Tbsp cocoa powder

Place everything in a blender and blend.

Hot Mexican Hot Chocolate

A spicy, healthier hot chocolate.

1 ¼ cup plain soy, almond, rice or hemp milk
2 Tbsp cocoa powder, dark
¼ tsp cayenne powder, less, or more, to taste
2 pinches of cinnamon powder
pinch of chili powder
2 tsp dark cane sugar, or dark maple syrup

Serves one.

Place everything in a pot and heat.

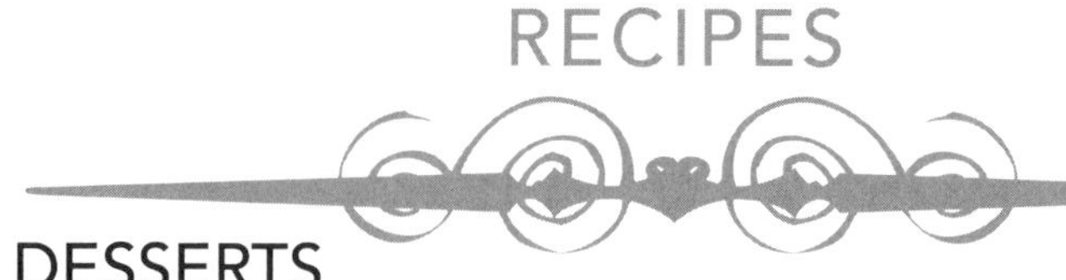

DESSERTS

Chocolate Tea

A great healthy and delicious beverage loaded in antioxidants.

1 rounded tsp of high quality green tea leaves

1 tsp-Tbsp of cocoa nibs, depends on how chocolaty you like it

---

Place both the green tea and the cocoa nibs in mesh tea holder, in a cup, and pour boiling water over them.

Cover, and let stand for about 10 minutes, or longer.

Drink.

Chocolate Coffee

A great antioxidant rich delicious drink. Serves two.

- 2 ½ small Greek coffee cups of water
- 2 well rounded tsp of Greek coffee
- 2 tsp of dark maple syrup
- ¼ tsp cinnamon, more if you like
- 2-3 tsp of cocoa powder, more if you like

In a Greek coffee pot, place the water, using 2 ½ Greek coffee cups as the measure of a cup, the Greek coffee, the maple syrup, the cinnamon, and the cocoa powder.

Stir.

Bring to a boil, stirring now and then, and watching it (it boils over quickly), then quickly remove from the heat before it boils over, stir, and place it back on the heat, very briefly, remove as it froths up.

Repeat 3 times.

Serve by pouring into the Greek coffee cups.

Let it settle, and drink, leaving the coffee on the bottom of the cups.

CHAPTER 2 REFERENCES

1. Havsteen B. Flavonoids, a class of natural products of high pharmacological potency. *Biochem Pharmacol* 1983;32:1141-8.

2. Middleton E. The flavonoids. *Trend Pharmaceut Sci* 1984;5:335-8.

3. Casini ML, Marelli G, Papaleo E, *et al.* Psychological assessment of the effects of treatment with phytoestrogens on postmenopausal women: a randomized, double-blind, crossover, placebo-controlled study. *Fertil Steril* 2006;85:972-8.

4. Albertazzi P, Pansini F. The effect of dietary soy supplementation on hot flashes. *Obstet Gynecol* 1998;91:6-11.

5. Han KK, *et al.* Benefits of soy isoflavone therapeutic regimen on menopausal symptoms. *Obstet Gynecol* 2002;99:389-94.

6. Faure ED, *et al.* Effects of a standardized soy extract on hot flushes: a multicenter, double-blind, randomized, placebo-controlled study. *Menopause* 2002;9:329-34.

7. Chi X-X, Zhang T. The effects of soy isoflavone on bone density in north region of climacteric Chinese women. *J Clin Biochem Nutr* 2013;53:102-7.

8. Carmignani LO, Pedro AO, Costa-Paiva LH, *et al. Maturitas* 2010;67:262-9.

9. Shu XO, *et al.* Soy food intake and breast cancer survival. *JAMA* 2009;302:2473-43.

10. *PLoS One* 2013;8(11);e81968doi:10.1371/journal.pone.0081968.

11. Potter SM, *et al.* Soy protein and isofavones: their effects on blood lipids and bone density in postmenopausal women. *Am J Clin Nutr* 1998;68:1375-9S.

12. Alekel DL, *et al.* Isoflavone-rich soy protein isolate attenuates bone loss in the lumbar spine of perimenopausal women. *Am J Clin Nutr* 2000;72:844-52.

13. Zhang X, *et al.* Prospective cohort study of soy food consumption and risk of bone fracture among postmenopausal women. *Arch Intern Med* 2005;165:1890-95.

14. Chi X-X, Zhang T. The effects of soy isoflavone on bone density in north region of climacteric Chinese women. *J Clin Biochem Nutr* 2013;53:102-7.

15. Wadworth AN, Faulds D. Hydroxyethylruosides: a review of its pharmacology, and therapeutic efficacy in venous insufficiency and related disorders. *Drug* 1992;44:1013-32.

16. Sohn C, Jahnichen C, Bastert G. Effectiveness of beta-hydroxyethylrutoside in patients with varicose veins in pregnancy. *Zentralbl Gynakol* 1995;117:190-7.

17. Sinnatamby CS. The treatment of hemorrhoids. Role of hydroxyethylrutosides, troxerutin (Paroven; Varmoid; Venoruton). *Clin Trials* J 1973;2:45-50.

18. Clyne MB, Freeling P, Ginsborg S. Troxerutin in the treatment of haemorrhoids. *Practitioner* 1967;198:420-3.

19. Annoni F, Boccasanta P, Chiurazzi D, *et al.* Treatment of acute symptoms of hemorrhoid disease with high-dose oral O-(beta-hydroxyethyl)-rutosides. *Minerva Med* 1986;77:1663-8.

20. Wijayanegara H, Mose JC, Achmad L, *et al.* A clinical trial of hydroxyethylrutosides in the treatment of haemorrhoids of pregnancy. *J Int Med Res* 1992;20:54-60.

21. Rehn D, Brunnauer H, Diebschlag W, *et al.* Investigation of the therapeutic equivalence of different galenical preparations of O-(s-hydroxyethyl)-rutosides following multiple dose per oral administration. *Arzneimforsch* 1996;46:488-92.

22. Bergqvist D, Hallbook T, Lindblad B, *et al.* A double-blind trial of O-(s-hydroxyethyl)-rutoside in patients with chronic venous insufficiency. *Vasa* 1981;10:253-60.

23. Poynard T, Valterio C. Meta-analysis of hydroxyethylrutosides in the treatment of chronic venous insufficiency. *Vasa* 1994;23:244-50.

24. Unkauf M, Rehn D, Klinger J, *et al.* Investigation of the efficacy of oxerutins compared to placebo in patients with chronic venous insufficiency treated with compression stockings. *Arzneimforsch* 1996;46:478-82.

25. Wadworth AN, Faulds D. Hydroxyethylrutosides: a review of its pharmacology, and therapeutic efficacy in venous insufficiency and related disorders. *Drugs* 1992;44:1013-32.

26. Boisseau MR, Taccoen A, Garreau C, *et al.* Fibrinolysis and hemorheology in chronic venous insufficiency: a double blind study of troxerutin efficiency. *J Cardiovasc Surg* 1995;36:369-74.

27. Neumann HA, van den Broek MJ. A comparative clinical trial of graduated compression stockings and O-(beta-hydroxyethyl)-rutosides (HR) in the treatment of patients with chronic venous insufficiency. *Z Lymphol* 1995;19:8-11.

28. Renton S, Leon M, Belcaro G, *et al.* The effect of hydroxyethylrutosides on capillary filtration in moderate venous hypertension: a double blind study. *Int Angiol* 1994;13:259-62.

29. MacLennan WJ, Wilson J, Rattenhuber V, *et al.* Hydroxyethylrutosides in Elderly Patients with Chronic Venous Insufficiency: Its Efficacy and Tolerability. *Gerontology* 1994;40:45-52.

30. Lamson DW, Brignall MS. Antioxidants and cancer, part 3: quercetin. *Alt Med Rev* 2000;5:196-208.

31. Yang CS, Landau JM, Huang MT, *et al.* Inhibition of carcinogenesis by dietary polyphenolic compounds. *Annu Rev Nutr* 2001;21:381-406.

32. Ho C, *et al.* Antioxidative effect of polyphenol extract prepared from various Chinese teas. *Prev Med* 1992;21:520-5.

33. Li N, Sun Z, Han C, *et al.* The chemopreventive effects of tea on human oral precancerous mucosa lesions. *Proc Soc Exp Biol Med* 1999;220:218-24.

34. Yu GP, Hsieh CC, Wang LY, *et al.* Green-tea consumption and risk of stomach cancer: a population-based case-control study in Shanghai, China. *Cancer Causes & Control* 1995;6:532-8.

35. Hyunseok K, Sun YR, Kyung WO, *et al.* Green tea consumption and stomach cancer risk: a meta-analysis. *Epidemiol Health* 2010;doi:10.4178/eouh/e2010001.

36. Gao YT, McLaughlin JK, Blot WJ, *et al.* Reduced risk of esophageal cancer associated with green tea consumption. *J Natl Cancer Inst* 1994;86:855-8.

37. *Carcinogenesis* 2002.

38. Blot WJ, Chow WH, McLaughlin JK. Tea and cancer: a review of the epidemiological evidence. *Eur J Cancer Prev* 1996;5:425-38.

39. Ji BT, Chow WH, Hsing AW, *et al.* Green tea consumption and the risk of pancreatic and colorectal cancers. *Int J Cancer* 1997;70:255-8.

40. Fujiki H. Two stages of cancer prevention with green tea. *J Cancer Res Clin Oncol* 1999;125:589-97.

41. Yang G, Shu XO, Li H, *et al.* Prospective cohort study of green tea consumption and colorectal cancer risk in women. *Cancer Epidemiol Biomarkers Prev* 2007;16:1219-23.

42. Ohno Y, Wakai K, Genka K, *et al.* Tea consumption and lung cancer risk: A case-control study in Okinawa, Japan. *Jpn J Cancer Res* 1995;86:1027-34.

43. Nakachi K, Suemasu K, Suga K, *et al.* Influence of drinking green tea on breast cancer malignancy among Japanese patients. *Cancer Science* 1998;89:254-261.

44. Fujiki H. Two stages of cancer prevention with green tea. *J Cancer Res Clin Oncol* 1999;125:589-97.

45. Wu AH, Yu MC, Tseng CC, *et al.* Green tea and risk of breast cancer in Asian Americans. *Int J Cancer* 2003;106:574-9.

46. Paschka AG, Butler R, Young CY. Induction of apoptosis in prostate cancer cell lines by the green tea component, (-)-epigallocatechin-3-gallate. *Cancer Letters* 1998;130:1-7.

47. Berttuzzi S, Brausi M, Rizzi F, *et al.* Chemoprevention of human prostate cancer by oral administration of green tea catechins in volunteers with high-grade prostate intraepithelial neoplasia: a preliminary report from a one year proof-of-principle study. *Cancer Res* 2006;66:1234-40.

48. Kono S, *et al.* Green tea consumption and serum lipid profiles: a cross-sectional study in Northern Kyushu, Japan. *Prev Med* 1992;21:526-31.

49. Sagesaka-Mitane Y, Milwa M, Okada S. Platelet aggregation inhibitors in hot water extract of green tea. *Chem Pharm Bull* 1990;38:790-93.

50. Stensvold I, *et al.* Tea consumption. Relationship to cholesterol, blood pressure, and coronary and total mortality. *Prev Med* 1992;21:546-53.

51. Imai K, Nakachi K. Cross sectional study of effects of drinking green tea on cardiovascular and liver diseases. *BMJ* 1995;310:693-96.

52. Kono S, *et al.* Green tea consumption and serum lipid profiles: a cross-sectional study in northern Kyushu, Japan. *Prev Med* 1992;21:526-31.

53. Nantz MP, Rowe CA, Bukowski JF, *et al.* Standardized capsule of Camellia sinensis lowers cardiovascular risk factors in a randomized, double-blind, placebo-controlled study. *Nutrition* 2009;25:147-54.

54. Sato Y, Nakatsuka H, Watanabe T, *et al.* Possible contribution of green tea drinking habits to the prevention of stroke. *Tohuku Journal of Experimental Medicine* 1989;157:337-43.

55. Bogdanski P, Suliburska J, Szulinska M, *et al.* Green tea extract reduces blood pressure, inflammatory biomarkers, and oxidative stress and improves parameters associated with insulin resistance in obese, hypertensive patients. *Nutr Res* 2012;32:421-7.

56. Otakes S, Maakimura M, Kuroki T, *et al.* Anticaries effects of polyphenolic compounds from Japanese green tea. *Caries Research* 1991;25:438-443.

57. Wu CD, Wei GX. Tea as a functional food for oral health. *Nutrition* 2002;18:443–4.

58. Makimura M, Hirasawa M, Kobayashi K, *et al.* Inhibitory effect of tea catechins on collagenase activity. *J Periodontol* 1993;64:630-36.

59. Sakanaka S, Aizawa M, Kim M, *et al.* Inhibitory effects of green tea polyphenols on growth and cellular adherence of an oral bacterium, *Porphyromonas gingivalis. Biosci Biotech Biochem* 1996;60:745-49..

60. Hirasawa M, Takada K, Makimura M, *et al.* Improvement of periodontal status by green tea catechin using a local deliver system: A clinical study *Journal of Periodontal Research* 2002;37:433-438.

61. Jenabian N, Moghadamnia AA, Karami E, *et al.* The effect of *Camellia sinensis* (green tea) mouthwash on plaque-induced gingivitis: a single-blinded randomized controlled clinical trial. *Daru* 2012;20:39.doi:10.1186/2008-2231-20-39.

62. Gomez Trillo JT. Varicose veins of the lower extremities. Symptomatic treatment with a new vasculotrophic agent. *Prensa Med Mex* 1973;38:293-6.

63. Royer RJ, Schmidt CL. Evaluation of venotropic drugs by venous gas plethysmography. A study of procyanidolic oligomers. *Sem Hop* 1981;57:2009-13.

64. Delacroix P. Etude en Double Avengle de l'Endotelon dans l'Insuffisance Veineuse Chronique. *Therapeutique, la Revue de Medicine* 1981;27-28:1793-1802.

65. Thebaut JF, Thebaut P, Vin F. Study of Endotelon in functional manifestations of peripheral venous insufficiency. *Gazette Medicale* 1985;92:96-100.

66. Teglio L, Mazzanti C, Tronconi R, *et al. Vaccinium myrtillus* anthocyanosides (Tegens) in the treatment of venous insufficiency of lower limbs and acute piles in pregnancy. *Quaderni di Clinica Osterica e Ginecologica* 1987;42:221-31.

67. Henriet JP. Veno-lymphatic insufficiency: 4,729 patients undergoing hormonal and procyanidol oligomer therapy. *Phlebologie* 1993;46:313-325.

1. Fisher N, Hughes M, Gerhard-Herman M. Flavanol-rich cocoa induces nitric oxide-dependent vasodilation in healthy humans. *J Hypertens* 2003;21:2281-2286.

2. Engler MB, Engler M, Chen C, *et al.* Flavonoid-rich dark chocolate improves endothelial function and increases plasma epicatechin concentrations in healthy adults. *J Am Coll Nutr* 2004;23:197-204.

3. Taubert D, Berkels R, Roesen R, *et al.* Chocolate and blood pressure in the elderly individuals with isolated systolic hypertension. *JAMA* 2003;29:1029-1030.

4. Ding E, Hutfless S, Ding X, Girotra S. Chocolate and prevention of cardiovascular disease: a systematic review *Nutr & Metabol* 2006;3:1-12.

5. Djoussé L, *et al.* Chocolate consumption is inversely associated with prevalent coronary heart disease: the National Heart, Lung, and Blood Institute Family Heart Study. *Clin Nutr* 2010; [epub ahead of print]. doi:10.1016/j.clnu.2010.08.005.

6. Chun Shing Kwok, S Matthijs Boekholdt, Marleen A H Lentjes, *et al.* Habitual chocolate consumption and risk of cardiovascular disease among healthy men and women. *Heart* 2015;doi: 10.1136/heartjnl-2014-307050

7. Djoussé L, *et al.* Chocolate consumption is inversely associated with calcified atherosclerotic plaque in the coronary arteries: the NHLBI family heart study. *Clin Nutr* 2010; [epub ahead of print]. doi:10.1016/j.clnu.2010.06.011.

8. Janszky I, Mukamal KJ, Ljung R, *et. al.* Chocolate consumption and mortality following a first acute myocardial infarction: the Stockholm Heart Epidemiology Program. *J Intern Med* 2009;266:248-257.

9. Ding E, Hutfless S, Ding X, Girotra S. Chocolate and prevention of cardiovascular disease: a systematic review *Nutr & Metabol* 2006;3:1-12.

10. Khawaja O, Gaziano JM, Djoussé L. Chocolate and coronary heart disease: a systematic review. *Curr Atheroscler Rep* 2011 Sep 6; [Epub ahead of print]. doi: 10.1007/s11883-011-0203-2.

11. Buitrago-Lopez A, et al. Chocolate consumption and cardiometabolic disorders: systematic review and meta-analysis. *BMJ* 2011;343:d4488doi:10.1136/bmj.d4488.

12. Buijsse B, Feskens EJ, Kok FJ, *et al.* Cocoa intake, blood pressure, and cardiovascular mortality: the Zutphen Elderly Study. *Arch Intern Med* 2006;166:411-417.

13. Buijsse B, *et al.* Chocolate consumption in relation to blood pressure and risk of cardiovascular disease in German adults. *Eur Heart J* 2010 [Epub ahead of print]. doi:10.1093/eurheartj/ehq068.

14. Chun Shing Kwok, S Matthijs Boekholdt, Marleen A H Lentjes, *et al.* Habitual chocolate consumption and risk of cardiovascular disease among healthy men and women. *Heart* 2015;doi: 10.1136/heartjnl-2014-307050.

15. Larsson SC, Virtamo J, Wolk A. Chocolate Consumption and Risk of Stroke in Women. *J Am Coll Cardiol* 2011;doi:10.1016/j.jacc.2011.07.023.

16. Jia-Yi Dong, Hiroyasu Iso, Kazumasa Yamagishi, *et al.* Chocolate consumption and risk of stroke among men and women: A large population-based, prospective cohort study. *Atherosclerosis* 2017;260:8-12

17. Larsson SC, Virtamo J, Wolk A. Chocolate consumption and risk of stroke: A prospective cohort of men and meta-analysis. *Neurology* 2012;79:1223-29.

18. Buitrago-Lopez A, *et al.* Chocolate consumption and cardiometabolic disorders: systematic review and meta-analysis. *BMJ* 2011;343:d4488doi:10.1136/bmj.d4488.

19. Janszky I, Mukamal KJ, Ljung R *et al.* Chocolate consumption and mortality following a first acute myocardial infarction: the Stockholm Heart Epidemiology Program. *J Intern Med* 2009;266:248-57.

1. Baba S, *et al.* Plasma LDL and HDL cholesterol and oxidized LDL concentrations are altered in normo- and hypercholesterolemic humans after intake of different levels of cocoa powder. *J Nutr* 2007;137:1436-41.

2. Wilson PWF. High-density lipoprotein, low-density lipoprotein and coronary artery disease. *Am J Cardiol* 1990;66:7A-10A.

3. Hamed MS, *et al.* Dark chocolate effect on platelet activity, C-reactive protein and lipid profile: a pilot study. *South Med J* 2008;101:1203-8.

4. Balzer J, Rassaf T, Heiss C, *et al.* Sustained benefits in vascular function through flavanol-containing cocoa in medicated diabetic patients: a double-masked, randomized, controlled trial. *J Am Coll Cardiol* 2008;51:2141-2149.

5. Grassi D, *et al.* Blood pressure is reduced and insulin sensitivity increased in glucose-intolerant, hypertensive subjects after 15 days of consuming high-polyphenol dark chocolate. *J Nutr* 2008;138:1671-6.

6. Khawaja O, Gaziano JM, Djoussé L. Chocolate and coronary heart disease: a systematic review. *Curr Atheroscler Rep* 2011 Sep 6; [Epub ahead of print]. doi: 10.1007/s11883-011-0203-2.

7. Hooper L, *et al.* Effects of chocolate, cocoa, and flavan-3-ols on cardiovascular health: a systematic review and meta-analysis of randomized trials. *Am J Clin Nutr* 2012;95:740-51.

8. Tokede OA, Gaziano JM, Djousse L. Effects of cocoa products/dark chocolate on serum lipids: a meta-analysis. *European Journal of Clinical Nutrition* 2011;65:879-886.

9. Zomer E, *et al.* The effectiveness and cost effectiveness of dark chocolate consumption as prevention therapy in people at high risk of cardiovascular disease: best case scenario analysis using a Markov model. *BMJ* 2012;344:e3657.

10. Hooper L, Kay C, Abdelhamid A, *et al.* Effects of chocolate, cocoa, and flavan-3-ols on cardiovascular health: a systematic review and meta-analysis of randomized trials. *Am J Clin Nutr* 2012 Mar;95:740-751.

11. Arranz S, Valderas-Martinez P, Chiva-Blanch G, *et al.* Cardioprotective effects of cocoa: Clinical evidence from randomized clinical intervention trials in humans. *Mol Nutr Food Res* 2013;57:936-947.

12. Nanetti L, *et al.* Effect of consumption of dark chocolate on lipoproteins and serum lipids. *Mediterranean Journal of Nutrition and Metabolism* 2008;1:25-31.

13. Wan Y, *et al.* Effects of cocoa powder and dark chocolate on LDL oxidative susceptibility and prostaglandin concentrations in humans. *Am Soc Clin Nutr* 2001;74:596-602.

14. Baba S, *et al.* Plasma LDL and HDL cholesterol and oxidized LDL concentrations are altered in normo- and hypercholesterolemic humans after intake of different levels of cocoa powder. *J Nutr* 2007;137:1436-41.

15. Nanetti L, *et al.* Effect of consumption of dark chocolate on oxidative stress in lipoproteins and platelets in women and in men. *Appetite* 2012;58:400-405.

16. Shrime MG, Bauer SR, McDonald AC, *et al.* Flavonoid-rich cocoa consumption affects multiple cardiovascular risk factors in a meta-analysis of short-term studies. *J Nutr* 2011;141:1982-1988.

17. Wan, Y, *et al.* Effects of cocoa powder and dark chocolate on LDL oxidative susceptibility and prostaglandin concentrations in humans. *American Society for Clinical Nutrition* 2001;74:596-602.

18. Mursu J, *et al.* Dark Chocolate Consumption Increases HDL Cholesterol Concentration and Chocolate Fatty Acids May Inhibit Lipid Peroxidation in Healthy Humans. *Free Radical Biology and Medicine* 2004;37:1351-9.

19. Wilson PWF. High-density lipoprotein, low-density lipoprotein and coronary artery disease. *Am J Cardiol* 1990;66:7A-10A.

20. Baba S, *et al.* Plasma LDL and HDL cholesterol and oxidized LDL concentrations are altered in normo- and hypercholesterolemic humans after intake of different levels of cocoa powder. *J Nutr* 2007;137:1436-41.

21. Hamed MS, *et al.* Dark chocolate effect on platelet activity, C-reactive protein and lipid profile: a pilot study. *South Med J* 2008;101:1203-8.

22. Monagas M, Khan N, Andres-Lacueva C, *et al.* Effect of cocoa powder on the modulation of inflammatory biomarkers in patients at high risk of cardiovascular disease. *Am J Clin Nutr* 2009;90:1144-1150.

23. Mellor DD, *et al.* High-cocoa polyphenol-rich chocolate improves HDL cholesterol in Type 2 diabetes patients. *Diabet Med* 2010;27:1318-21.

24. Khawaja O, Gaziano JM, Djoussé L. Chocolate and coronary heart disease: a systematic review. *Curr Atheroscler Rep* 2011 [Epub ahead of print]. doi: 10.1007/s11883-011-0203-2.

25. Tokede OA, Gaziano JM, Djousse L. Effects of cocoa products/dark chocolate on serum lipids: a meta-analysis. *European Journal of Clinical Nutrition* 2011;65:879-886.

26. Shrime MG, Bauer SR, McDonald AC, *et al.* Flavonoid-rich cocoa consumption affects multiple cardiovascular risk factors in a meta-analysis of short-term studies. *J Nutr* 2011;141:1982-1988.

27. Hooper L, *et al.* Effects of chocolate, cocoa, and flavan-3-ols on cardiovascular health: a systematic review and meta-analysis of randomized trials. *Am J Clin Nutr* 2012;95:740-51.

28. Arranz S, Valderas-Martinez P, Chiva-Blanch G, *et al.* Cardioprotective effects of cocoa: Clinical evidence from randomized clinical intervention trials in humans. *Mol Nutr Food Res* 2013;57:936-947.

29. Lin X, Zhang I, Li A, *et al.* Cocoa flavanol intake and biomarkers for cardiometabolic health: a systematic review and meta-analysis of randomized controlled trials. *J Nutr* 2016;146(11):2325-2333.

30. Martínez-López S, Sarriá B, Sierra-Cinos JL, *et al.* Realistic intake of a flavanol-rich soluble cocoa product increases HDL-cholesterol without inducing anthropometric changes in healthy and moderately hypercholesterolemic subjects. *Food Funct* 2014;5:364-374.

31. Neufingerl N, Zebregs YEMP, Schuring EAH, *et al.* Effect of cocoa and theobromine consumption on serum HDL-cholesterol concentrations: a randomized controlled trial. *Am J Clin Nutr* 2013;97:1201-1209.

32. Kromhout D, Menotti A, Bloemberg B, *et al.* Dietary saturated and trans fatty acids and cholesterol and 25-year mortality from coronary heart disease: the Seven Countries Study. *Prev Med* 1995;24:308-15.

33. Thorogood M, Carter R, Benfield L, *et al.* Plasma lipids and lipoprotein cholesterol concentrations in people with different diets in Britain. *Br Med J* (Clin Res Ed) 1987;295:351-3.

34. Resnicow K, Barone J, Engle A, *et al.* Diet and serum lipids in vegan vegetarians: a model for risk reduction. *J Am Dietet Assoc* 1991;91:447-53.

35. Ripsin CM, Keenan JM, Jacobs DR, *et al.* Oat products and lipid lowering—a meta-analysis. *JAMA*1992;267:3317-25.

36. Romero A L, *et al.* Cookies enriched with psyllium or oat bran lower plasma LDL cholesterol in normal and hypercholesterolemic men from Northern Mexico. *J Am Coll Nutr* 1998;17:601-08.

37. Uusitupa M I, Ruuskanen E, Mäkinen E *et al.* A controlled study on the effect of beta-glucan-rich oat bran on serum lipids in hypercholesterolemic subjects: relation to apolipoprotein E phenotype. *J Am Coll Nutr* 1992;11:651-59.

38. Braaten J T, Wood PJ, Scott FW, *et al.* Oat beta-glucan reduces blood cholesterol concentration in hypercholesterolemic subjects. *Eur J Clin Nutr* 1994;48:465-74.

39. Davidson M H, *et al.* The hypocholesterolemic effects of beta-glucan in oatmeal and oat bran. A dose-controlled study. *JAMA* 1991;265:1833-39.

40. Bierenbaum ML, Reichstein R, Watkins TR. Reducing atherogenic risk in hyperlipemic humans with flaxseed supplementation: a preliminary report. *J Am Coll Nutr* 1993;12:501-4.

41. Cunnane SC, Ganguli S, Menard C, *et al.* High alpha-linolenic acid flaxseed *(Linum usitatissimum)*: some nutritional properties in humans. *Br J Nutr* 1993;69:443-53.

42. Arjmandi BH, Khan DA, Juma S, *et al.* Whole flaxseed consumption lowers serum LDL-cholesterol and lipoprotein(a) concentrations in postmenopausal women. *Nutr Res* 1998;18:1203-14.

43. Pan A, *et al.* Meta-analysis of the effects of flaxseed interventions on blood lipids. *Am J Clin Nutr* 2009;90:288-97.

44. Romero A L, Romero JE, Falaviz S, *et al.* Cookies enriched with psyllium or oat bran lower plasma LDL cholesterol in normal and hypercholesterolemic men from Northern Mexico. *J Am Coll Nutr* 1998;17:601-08.

45. Anderson JW, Allgood LD, Lawrence A, *et al.* Cholesterol-lowering effects of psyllium intake adjunctive to diet therapy in men and women with hypercholesterolemia: meta-analysis of 8 controlled trials. *Am J Clin Nutr* 2000;71:472-9.

46. Anderson JW, Davidson MH, Blonde L, *et al.* Long-term cholesterol-lowering effects as an adjunct to diet therapy in the treatment of hypercholesterolemia. *Am J Clin Nutr* 2000;71:1433-8.

47. Olson BH, Anderson SM, Becker MP, *et al.* Psyllium-enriched cereals lower blood total cholesterol and LDL cholesterol, but not HDL cholesterol, in hypercholesterolemic adults: Results of a meta-analysis. *J Nutr*1997;127:1973-80.

48. Miettinen TA, Tarpila S. Effect of pectin on serum cholesterol, fecal bile acids and biliary lipids in normolipidemic and hyperlipidemic individuals. *Clin Chim Acta* 1977;79:471-7.

49. Walsh DE, Yaghoubian V, Behforooz A. Effect of glucomannan on obese patients: a clinical study. *Int J Obes* 1984;8:289-93.

50. Zhang MY, Huang CY, Wang X, *et al.* The effect of foods containing refined Konjac meal on human lipid metabolism. *Biomed Environ Sci* 1990;3:99-105.

51. Arvill A, Bodin L. Effect of short-term ingestion of konjac glucomannan on serum cholesterol in healthy men. *Am J Clin Nutr* 1995;61:585-9.

52. Vuksan V, Jenkins DJ, Spadafora P, *et al.* Konjac-mannan (glucomannan) improves glycemia and other associated risk factors for coronary heart disease in type 2 diabetes. A randomized controlled metabolic trial. *Diabetes Care* 1999;22:913-9.

53. Anderson, JW, Johnstone BM, Cook-Newell ME. Meta-analysis of the effects of soy protein intake on serum lipids. *N Engl J Med* 1995;3333:276-82.

54. Baum J A, *et al.* Long-term intake of soy protein improves blood lipid profiles and increases mononuclear cell low-density-lipoprotein receptor messenger RNA in hypercholesterolemic, postmenopausal women. *Am J Clin Nutr* 1998;68:545-51.

55. Crouse J R, 3rd, *et al.* A randomized trial comparing the effect of casein with that of soy protein containing varying amounts of isoflavones on plasma concentrations of lipids and lipoproteins. *Arch Intern Med* 1999;159:2070-76.

56. Sirtori CR, *et al.* Double-blind study of the addition of high-protein soya milk v. cows' milk to the diet of patients with severe hypercholesterolaemia and resistance to or intolerance of statins. *Br J Nutr* 1999;82:91-96.

57. Teixeira SR, *et al.* Effects of feeding 4 levels of soy protein for 3 and 6 wk on blood lipids and apolipoproteins in moderately hypercholesterolemic men. *Am J Clin Nutr* 2000;71:1077-84.

58. Sabaté J, Oda K, Ros E. Nut Consumption and Blood Lipid Levels: A Pooled Analysis of 25 Intervention Trials. *Arch Intern Med* 2010;170:821-27.

59. Sabaté J, Fraser GE, Burke K, *et al.* Effects of walnuts on serum lipid levels and blood pressure in normal men. *N Engl J Med* 1993;328:603-07.

60. Zambon D, *et al.* Effects of walnuts on the serum lipid profile of hypercholesterolemic subjects: the Barcelona Walnut Trial. *FASEB J* 1998;12:A506.

61. Zambon D, Sabaté J, Muñoz S, *et al.* Substituting walnuts for monounsaturated fat improves the serum lipid profile of hypercholesterolemic men and women. A randomized crossover trial. *Ann Intern Med* 2000;132:538-46.

62. Almrio RU, Vonghavaravat V, Wong R, V *et al.* Effects of walnut consumption on plasma fatty acids and lipoproteins in combined hyperlipidemia. *Am J Clin Nutr* 2001;74:72-79.

63. Spiller GA, Jenkins DJ, Cragen LN *et al.* Effect of a diet high in monounsaturated fat from almonds on plasma cholesterol and lipoproteins. *J Am Coll Nutr* 1992;11:126-30.

64. Spiller GA, Jenkins DAJ, Bosello O, *et al.* Nuts and plasma lipids: an almond-based diet lowers LDL-C while preserving HDL-C. *J Am Coll Nutr* 1998; 17:285-90.

65. Jambazian PR, *et al.* Almonds in the diet simultaneously improve plasma alpha-tocopherol concentrations and reduce plasma lipids. *J Am Dietetic Association* 2005;105:449-54.

66. Durak I, Köksal I, Kaçmaz M, *et al.* Hazelnut supplementation enhances plasma antioxidant potential and lowers plasma cholesterol levels. *Clin Chim Actia* 1999;284:113-15 [letter].

67. Edwards K, Kwaw I, Matud J, *et al.* Effect of pistachio nuts on serum lipid levels in patients with moderate hypercholesterolemia. *J Am Coll Nutr* 1999;18:229-32.

68. Chen P R, Chien KL, Su TC, *et al.* Dietary sesame reduces serum cholesterol and enhances antioxidant capacity in hypercholesterolemia. *Nutrition Research* 2005;25:559-67.

69. Wu WH, Kang YP, Wang NH *et al.* Sesame ingestion affects sex hormones, antioxidant status, and blood lipids in postmenopausal women. *J Nutr* 2006;136:1270-75.

70. Illingworth DR, Stein EA, Mitchel YB, *et al.* Comparative effects of lovastatin and niacin in primary hypercholesterolemia. *Arch Intern Med* 1994;154:1586-95.

71. Guyton JR, Blazing MA, Hagar J, *et al.* Extended-release niacin vs gemfibrozil for the treatment of low levels of high-density lipoprotein cholesterol. Niaspan-Gemfibrozil Study Group. *Arch Intern Med* 2000;160:1177-84.

72. Vega GL, Grundy SM. Lipoprotein responses to treatment with lovastatin, gemfibrozil, and nicotinic acid in normolipidemic patients with hypoalphalipoproteinemia. *Arch Intern Med* 1994;154:73-82.

73. Taylor AJ, Villnes TC, Stanek EJ, *et al.* Extended-release niacin or ezetimibe and carotid intima-media thickness. *N Engl J Med* 2009;361:2113-22.

74. Welsh A L., Ede M. Inositol hexaniocotinate for improved nicotinic acid therapy. *Int Record Med* 1961;174:9-15.

75. El-Enein, AMA, *et al.* The role of nicotinic acid and inositol hexaniacinate as anticholesterolemic and antilipemic agents. *Nutr Rep Intl* 1983;28:899-911.

76. Sunderland GT, Belch JJF, Sturrock RD, *et al.* A double-blind randomized placebo controlled trial of hexopal in primary Raynaud's disease. *Clin Rheumatol* 1988;7:46-49.

77. Agarwal RC, Singh SP, Saran RK, *et al.* Clinical trial of gugulipid new hypolipidemic agent of plant origin in primary hyperlipidemia. *Indian J Med Res* 1986;84:626-34.

78. Nityanand S, Srivastava JS, Asthana OP. Clinical trials with Gugulipid—a new hypolipidemic agent. *J Assoc Phys India* 1989; 37:323-8.

79. Singh RB, Niaz MA, Ghosh S. Hypolipidemic and antioxidant effects of Commiphora mukul as an adjunct to dietary therapy in patients with hypercholesterolemia. *Cardiovasc Drugs Ther* 1994;8:659-64.

80. Tripathi SN, Upadhyay BN. A clinical trial of Commiphora mukul in the patients of ischemic heart disease. *Journal of Molecular and Cellular Cardiology* 1878:10(Supp 1):124.

81. Wang J, Lu Z, Chi J, *et al.* Multicenter clinical trial of the serum lipid-lowering effects of a Monascus purpureus (red yeast) rice preparation from traditional Chinese medicine. *Curr Ther Res* 1997;58:964-78.

82. Heber D, Yip I, Ashley JM, *et al.* Cholesterol-lowering effects of a proprietary Chinese red-yeast-rice dietary supplement. *Am J Clin Nutr* 1999;69:231-36.

83. Rippe J, Bonovich K, Colfer C. A multi-center, self-controlled study of Cholestinin subjects with elevated cholesterol. 39th Annual Conference on Cardiovascular Disease Epidemiology and Prevention. Orlando, FL, 1999; March 24;27:1123.

84. Becker DJ, Gordon RY, Halbert SC, *et al.* Red yeast Rice for Dyslipidemia in Statin-Intolerant Patients: A Randomized Trial. *Ann Intern Med* 2009;150:830-39.

85. Liu J, Zhang J, Shi Y, *et al.* Chinese red yeast rice (Monascus purpureus) for primary hyperlipidemia: a meta-analysis of randomized controlled trials. *Chin Med* 2006;1:4.

86. Zeng T, Guo FF, Zhang Cl, *et al.* A meta-analysis of randomized, double-blind, placebo-controlled trials for the effects of garlic on serum lipid profiles. *J Sci Food Agric* 2012;92:1892-902.

87. Ried K, Toben C, Fakler P. Effect of garlic on serum lipids: an updated meta-analysis. *Nutr Rev* 2013;71:282-99.

88. Arsenio L, Bodria P, Magnati G, *et al.* Effectiveness of long-term treatment with pantethine in patients with dyslipidemia. *Clin Ther* 1986;8:537-45.

89. Prisco D, Rogasi PG, Matucci M, *et al.* Effect of oral treatment with pantethine on platelet and plasma phospholipids in IIa hyperlipoproteinemia. *Angiology* 1987;38:241-7.

90. Gaddi A, Descovich GC, Noseda G, *et al.* Controlled evaluation of pantethine, a natural hypolipidemic compound, in patients with different forms of hyperlipoproteinemia. *Atherosclerosis* 1984;50:73-83.

91. Rumberger JA, Napolitano J, Azumano I, *et al.* Pantethine, a derivative of vitamin B5 used as a nutritional supplement, favorably alters low-density lipoprotein cholesterol metabolism in low- to moderate-cardiovascular risk North American subjects: a triple-blinded placebo and diet-controlled investigation. *Nutr Res* 2011;31:608-15.

92. Evans M, Rumberger JA, Azumano I, *et al.* Pantethine, a derivative of vitamin B5, favorably alters total, LDL and non-HDL cholesterol in low to moderate cardiovascular risk subjects eligible for statin therapy: a triple-blinded placebo and diet-controlled investigation. *Vasc Health Risk Manag* 2014;10:89–100.

93. Simon JA. Vitamin C and cardiovascular disease: a review. *J Am Coll Nutr* 1992;11:107-27.

94. Gatto LM, Hallen GK, Brown AJ, *et al.* Ascorbic acid induces a favorable lipoprotein profile in women. J *Am Coll Nutr* 1996;15;154-58.

95. Frei B. Ascorbic acid protects lipids in human plasma and low-density lipoprotein against oxidative damage. *Am J Clin Nutr* 1991;54:1113-8S.

96. Belcher JD, Balla J, Balla G, *et al.* Vitamin E, LDL, and endothelium: Brief oral vitamin supplementation prevents oxidized LDL-mediated vascular injury in vitro. *Arterioscler Thromb* 1993;13:1779-89.

97. Kono S, Shinchi K, Ikeda N, *et al.* Green tea consumption and serum lipid profiles: a cross-sectional study in Northern Kyushu, Japan. *Prev Med* 1992;21:526-31.

98. Sagesaka-Mitane Y, Milwa M, Okada D. Platelet aggregation inhibitors in hot water extract of green tea. *Chem Pharm Bull* 1990;38:790-93.

99. Stensvold I, Tverdal A, Solvoll K, *et al.* Tea consumption. Relationship to cholesterol, blood pressure, and coronary and total mortality. *Prev Med* 1992;21:546-53.

100. Imai K, Nakachi K. Cross sectional study of effects of drinking green tea on cardiovascular and liver diseases. *BMJ* 1995;310:693-96.

101. Nutr Metab Cardio Dis 2012,doi:dx.doi.org/10.1016/j.numecd.2012.06.005.

102. Kong W, Wei J, Abidi P, *et al.* Berberine is a novel cholesterol-lowering drug working through a unique mechanism distinct from statins. *Nature Medicine* 2004;10:1344-1355.

103. Zhang Y, Li X, Zou D, *et al.* Treatment of type 2 diabetes and dyslipidemia with the natural plant alkaloid berberine. *JCEM* 2008;93:2559-65.

104. Yin J, Xing H, Ye J. Efficacy of berberine in patients with type 2 diabetes mellitus. *Metabolism* 2008;57:712-17.

105. Zhang H, Wei J, Xue R, *et al.* Berberine lowers blood glucose in type 2 diabetes mellitus patients through increasing insulin receptor expression. *Metabolism* 2010;59:285-92.

106. Englisch W, Beckers C, Unkauf M, *et al.* Efficacy of artichoke dry extract in patients with hyperlipoproteinemia. *Arzneimittelforschung* 2000;50:260-65.

107. Rondanelli M, Giacosa A, Opizzi A, *et al.* Beneficial effects of artichoke leaf extract supplementation on increasing HDL-cholesterol in subjects with primary mild hypercholesterolaemia: a double-blind, randomized, placebo-controlled trial. *Int J Food Sci Nutr* 2013;64:7-15.

108. Fintelmann V. Antidyspeptic and lipid-lowering effect of artichoke leaf extract. *Zeitschirfit fur Allgemeinmed* 1996;72:1-19.

1. Grassi D, *et al*. Short-term administration of dark chocolate is followed by a significant increase in insulin sensitivity and a decrease in blood pressure in healthy persons. *American Society for Clinical Nutrition* 2005;81:611-614.

2. di Giuseppe R, Di Castelnuovo A, Centritto F, *et al*. Regular consumption of dark chocolate is associated with low serum concentrations of C-reactive protein in a healthy Italian population. *J Nutr* 2008;138:1939-1945.

3. Al-Safi SA, Ayoub NM, Al-Doghim I, *et al*. Dark Chocolate and Blood Pressure: A Novel Study from Jordan. *Current Drug Delivery* 2011;8:595-9.

4. Ried K, Sullivan TR, Fakler P, *et al*. Effect of cocoa on blood pressure. *Cochrane Database Syst Rev*. August 15, 2012;8:CD008893.doi: 10.1002/14651858.CD008893.pub2.

5. Taubert D, Roesen R, Lehmann C, *et al*. Effects of low habitual cocoa intake on blood pressure and bioactive nitric oxide: a randomized controlled trial *JAMA* 2007;298:49-60.

6. Sudarma V, Sukmaniah S, Siregar P. Effect of dark chocolate on nitric oxide serum levels and blood pressure in prehypertension subjects. *Acta Med Indones* 2011;43:224-228.

7. Desch S, Kobler D, Schmidt J, *et al*. Low vs. Higher-Dose Dark Chocolate and Blood Pressure in Cardiovascular High-Risk Patients. *Am J Hypertens* 2010;23:694-700.

8. Taubert D, Berkels R, Roesen R, *et al*. Chocolate and blood pressure in elderly individuals with isolated systolic hypertension. *JAMA* 2003;290:1029-30.

9. Ried K, Sullivan T, Fakler P, *et al*. Does chocolate reduce blood pressure? A meta-analysis. *BMC Med* 2010;8:39. doi:10.1186/1741-7015-8-39.

10. Desch S, Schmidt J, Kobler D, *et al*. Effect of cocoa products on blood pressure: systematic review and meta-analysis. *Am J Hypertens* 2010;23:97-103.

11. Fernández-Murga L, Tarín JJ, García-Perez MA, *et al.* The impact of chocolate on cardiovascular health. *Maturitas* 2011;69:312-321.

12. Zomer E, Owen A, Magliano DJ, *et al.* The effectiveness and cost effectiveness of dark chocolate consumption as prevention therapy in people at high risk of cardiovascular disease: best case scenario analysis using a Markov model. *BMJ* 2012;344:e3657.

13. Buijsse B, Feskens EJ, Kok FJ, *et al.* Cocoa Intake, Blood Pressure, and Cardiovascular Mortality: the Zutphen Elderly Study. *Arch Intern Med* 2006;166:411–17.

14. Hooper L, Kroon PA, Rimm EB, *et al.* Flavonoids, flavonoid-rich foods, and cardiovascular risk: a meta-analysis of randomized controlled trials. *Am J Clin Nutr* 2008 Jul;88(1):38-50.

15. Khawaja O, Gaziano JM, Djoussé L. Chocolate and coronary heart disease: a systematic review. *Curr Atheroscler Rep* 2011;13:447-52.

16. Taubert D, Roesen R, Schomig E. Effect of cocoa and tea intake on blood pressure; a meta-analysis *Arch Intern Med* 2007;167:626-634.

17. Shrime MG, Bauer SR, McDonald AC, *et al.* Flavonoid-rich cocoa consumption affects multiple cardiovascular risk factors in a meta-analysis of short-term studies. *J Nutr* 2011;141:1982-1988.

18. Hooper L, Kay C, Abdelhamid A, *et al.* Effects of chocolate, cocoa, and flavan-3-ols on cardiovascular health: a systematic review and meta-analysis of randomized trials. *Am J Clin Nutr* 2012;95:740-751.

19. Ellinger S, Reusch A, Stehle P, *et al.* Epicatechin ingested via cocoa products reduces blood pressure in humans: a nonlinear regression model with a Bayesian approach. *Am J Clin Nutr* 2012;95:1365-1377.

20. Almoosawi S, Fyfe L, Ho C, *et al.* The effect of polyphenol-rich dark chocolate on fasting capillary whole blood glucose, total cholesterol, blood pressure and glucocorticoids in healthy overweight and obese subjects. *Br J Nutr* 2010;103:842-850.

21. Berry NM, Davison K, Coates AM, *et al.* Impact of cocoa flavanol consumption on blood pressure responsiveness to exercise. *Br J Nutr* 2010;103:1480-1484.

22. Muniyappa R,Hall G, Kolodziej TL, *et al.* Cocoa consumption for 2 wk enhances insulin-mediated vasodilatation without improving blood pressure or insulin resistance in essential hypertension. *Am J Clin Nutr* 2008;88:1685-96.

23. Reid K, Frank OR, Stocks NP. Dark chocolate or tomato extract for prehypertension: a randomised controlled trial. *BMC Complement Altern Med* 2009;8:9-22.

24. van den Bogaard B, Draijer R, Westerhof BE, *et al.* Effects on peripheral and central blood pressure of cocoa with natural or high-dose theobromine: a randomized, double-blind crossover trial. *Hypertension* 2010;56:839-846.

25. Martínez-López S, Sarriá B, Sierra-Cinos JL, *et al.* Realistic intake of a flavanol-rich soluble cocoa product increases HDL-cholesterol without inducing anthropometric changes in healthy and moderately hypercholesterolemic subjects. *Food Funct* 2014;5:364-374.

26. Rouse I L, Beilin LJ, Mahoney DP, *et al.* Vegetarian diet and blood pressure. *Lancet* 1983;ii:742-43.

27. Margetts BM, Beilin LJ, Vandongen R, *et al.* Vegetarian diet in mild hypertension: a randomised controlled trial. *BMJ* 1986;293:1468-71.

28. Rouse I L, Beilin LJ, Mahoney DP, *et al.* Vegetarian diet and blood pressure. *Lancet* 1983;ii:742-43.

29. McDougall J, Litzaue K, Haver E, *et al.* Rapid reduction of serum cholesterol and blood pressure by a twelve-day, very low fat, strictly vegetarian diet. *J Am Coll Nutr* 1995;14:491-96.

30. Lindahl O, Lindwall L, Spångberg A, *et al.* A vegan regimen with reduced medication in the treatment of hypertension. *Br J Nutr* 1984;52:11-20

31. Appel LJ, Moore TJ, Boarzanek E, *et al.* A clinical trial of the effects of dietary patterns on blood pressure. *N Engl J Med* 1997;336:1117-24.

32. Stamler J, Rose G, Elliott P, *et al.* Findings of the international cooperative IN-TERSALT study. *Hypertension* 1991;17(1 Suppl):I9-15.

33. MacGregor G A, Markandu ND, Sagnella GA, *et al.* Double-blind study of three sodium intakes and long-term effects of sodium restriction in essential hypertension. *Lancet* 1989;2:1244-47.

34. Cutler JA, Follmann D, Allender PS. Randomized trials of sodium reduction: an overview. *Am J Clin Nutr* 1997;65(Suppl):643S-51S.

35. Hajjar IM, Grim CE, George V, *et al.* Impact of diet on blood pressure and age-related changes in blood pressure in the U.S. population: Analysis of NHANES III. *Arch Intern Med* 2001;161:589-93.

36. Cappuccio FP, MacGregor GA. Does potassium supplementation lower blood pressure? A meta-analysis of published trials. *J Hypertens* 1991;9:465-73.

37. Kass L, Weekes J, Carpenter J. Effect of magnesium supplementation on blood pressure: a meta-analysis. *Eur J Clin Nutr* 2012;66:411-8.

38. Iaconon J M, Puska P, Dougherty RM, *et al.* Effect of dietary fat on blood pressure in a rural Finnish population. *Am J Clin Nutr* 1983;38:860-69.

39. Zheng, H-J, Folsom AR, Ma J, *et al.* Plasma fatty acid composition and 6-year incidence of hypertension in middle-aged adults. *Am J Epidemiol* 1999;150:492-500.

40. Rodriguez-Leyva D, Weighell W, Edel AL, *et al.* Potent Antihypertensive Action of Dietary Flaxseed in Hypertensive Patients. *Hypertension* 2013;62:1081-9.

41. Ferrara L A, Raimondi AS, d'Episcopo L, *et al.* Olive Oil and Reduced Need for Antihypertensive Medications. *Arch Intern Med* 2000;160:837-842.

42. Liu XX, Si SH, Chen JZ, *et al.* Effect of soy isoflavones on blood pressure: a meta-analysis of randomized controlled trials. *Nutr Metab Cardiovasc Dis* 2012;22:463-70.

43. Ness A R, Chee D, Elliott P. Vitamin C and blood pressure-an overview. *J Human Hypertens* 1998;16:925-32.

44. Juraschek SP, Guallar E, Appel LJ, *et al.* Effects of vitamin C supplementation on blood pressure: a meta-analysis of randomized controlled trials. *Am J Clin Nutr* 2012;95:1079-88.

45. Ayback M, Sermet A, Ayyildiz MO, *et al.* Effect of oral pyridoxine hydrochloride supplementation on arterial blood pressure in patients with essential hypertension. *Arzneim Forsch* 1995;45:1271-73.

46. Digiesi V, Cantini F, Brodbeck B. Effect of coenzyme Q10 on essential arterial hypertension. *Curr Ther Res* 1990;47:841-45.

47. Singh RB, Niaz MA, Rastogi SS, *et al.* Effect of hydrosoluble coenzyme Q10 on blood pressure and insulin resistance in hypertensive patients with coronary artery disease. *J Hum Hypertens* 1999;13:203-08.

48. Burke BE, Neuenschwander R, Olson RD. Randomized, double-blind, placebo-controlled trial of coenzyme Q10 in isolated systolic hypertension. *South Med J* 2001;94:1112-17.

49. Reid K, Frank OR, Stocks NP. Aged garlic extract reduces blood pressure in hypertensives: a dose-response trial. *Eur J Clin Nutr* 2013;67:64-70.

50. Ried K, Frank OR, Stocks NP, *et al.* Effect of garlic on blood pressure: a systematic review and meta-analysis. *BMC Cardiovasc Disord* 2008;8:13.

51. Cassidy A, O'Reilly ÉJ, Kay C, *et al.* Habitual intake of flavonoid subclass and incident hypertension in adults. *Am J Clin Nutr* 2011;1993:338-47.

52. McAnulty LS, Collier SR, Landram MJ, *et al.* Six weeks daily ingestion of whole blueberry powder increases natural killer cell counts and reduces arterial stiffness in sedentary males and females. *Nutr Res* 2014;34:577-84.

53. Robinson M, Lu B, Edirisinghe I, *et al.* Effect of grape seed extract on blood pressure in subjects with pre-hypertension. *J Pharm Nutr Sci* 2012:155-9.

54. Cherif S. A clinical trial of a titrated Olea extract in the treatment of essential arterial hypertension. *J Pharm Belg* 1996;51:69-71.

55. Susalit E, Agus N, Effendi I, *et al.* Olive (Olea europaea) leaf extract effective in patients with stage-1 hypertension: comparison with Captopril. *Phytomed* 2011;18:251-8.

56. Haji Faraji M, Haji Tarkhani AH. The effect of sour tea (Hibiscus sabdariffa) on essential hypertension. *J Ethnopharmacol* 1999;65:231-6.

57. McKay DL, Chen CY, Saltzman E, *et al.* Hibiscus sabdariffa L. tea (tisane) lowers blood pressure in prehypertensive and mildly hypertensive adults. *J Nutr* 2010;140:298-303.

58. Herrera-Arellano A, Flores-Romero S, Chavez-Soto MA, *et al.* Effectiveness and tolerability of a standardized extract from Hibiscus sabdariffa in patients with mild to moderate hypertension: a controlled and randomized clinical trial. *Phytomedicine* 2004;11:375-82.

59. Jin H, Zhang G, Cao X, *et al.* Treatment of hypertension by ling zhi combined with hypotensor and its effects on arterial, arteriolar and capillary pressure and microcirculation. Cited in Yarnell E, Abascal K, Hooper C. *Clinical Botanical Medicine.* Mary Ann Liebert: Larchmont NY 2002, p.74.

60. Asgary S, Naderi GH, Sarrafzadegan N, *et al.* Antihypertensive and antihy-perlipidemic effects of Achillea wilhelmsii. *Drugs Exp Clin Res* 2000;26:89-93.

1. Fisher N, Hughes M, Gerhard-Herman M. Flavanol-rich cocoa induces nitric oxide-dependent vasodilation in healthy humans. *Journal of Hypertension* 2003;21:2281-2286.

2. Engler MB, Engler M, Chen C, *et al.* Flavonoid-rich dark chocolate improves endothelial function and increases plasma epicatechin concentrations in healthy adults. *Journal of the American College of Nutrition* 2004;23:197-204.

3. Taubert D, Berkels R, Roesen R, *et al.* Chocolate and blood pressure in the elderly individuals with isolated systolic hypertension. *Journal of the American Medical Association* 2003;29:1029-1030.

4. Engler M, Engler M, Chen C, *et al.* Flavonoid-rich dark chocolate improves endothelial function and increases plasma epicatechin concetrations in healthy adults *J Am Coll Nutr* 2004;23(3):197-204.

5. Shrime MG, Bauer SR, McDonald AC, *et al.* Flavonoid-rich cocoa consumption affects multiple cardiovascular risk factors in a meta-analysis of short-term studies. *J Nutr* 2011;141:1982-1988.

6. Hooper L, Kroon PA, Rimm EB, *et al.* Flavonoids, flavonoid-rich foods, and cardiovascular risk: a meta-analysis of randomized controlled trials. *Am J Clin Nutr* 2008;88:38-50.

7. Schroeter H, Heiss C, Balzer J, *et al.* (-)-Epicatechin mediates beneficial effects of flavanol-rich cocoa on vascular function in humans. *PNAS* 2006;103:1024-1029.

8. Vlachopoulos C, Aznaouridis K, Alexopoulos N, *et al.* Effect of Dark Chocolate on Arterial Function in Healthy Individuals. *Am J Hypertension* 2005;18:785-91.

9. Pereira T, Maldonado J, Laranjeiro M, *et al.* Central arterial hemodynamic effects of dark chocolate ingestion in young healthy people: a randomized and controlled trial. *Cardiol Res Pract* 2014;2014:945951.

10. Westphal S, Luley C. Flavanol-rich cocoa ameliorates lipemia-induced endothelial dysfunction. *Heart Vessels* Dec 8, 2010; [epub ahead of print]. doi:10.1007/s00380-010-0085-1.

11. Shiina Y, Lee K, Kawakubo M, *et al.* Acute Effect of Oral Flavonoid-Rich Dark Chocolate Intake on Coronary Circulation by Transthoracic Doppler Echocardiography in Healthy Adults. *Circulation* 2007;116:11_369.

12. Shiina Y, Funabashi N, Lee K, *et al.* Acute effect of oral flavonoid-rich dark chocolate intake on coronary circulation, as compared with non-flavonoid white chocolate, by transthoracic Doppler echocardiography in healthy adults. *Int J Cardiol* 2009;131:424-9.

13. Heiss C, Sansone R, Karimi H, *et al.* Impact of cocoa flavanol intake on age-dependent vascular stiffness in healthy men: a randomized, controlled, double-masked trial. *Age* (Dordr) 2015;37(3):56.

14. Persson IAL, Persson K, Hägg S, *et al.* Effects of cocoa extract and dark chocolate on angiotensin-converting enzyme and nitric oxide in human endothelial cells and healthy volunteers - a nutrigenomics perspective. *J Cardiovasc Pharmacol* 2011;57:44-50.

15. Farouque HMO, Leung M, Hope S, *et al.* Acute and chronic effects of flavonol-rich cocoa on vascular function in subjects with coronary artery disease: a randomized double-blind placebo-controlled study. *Clin Sci* 2006;111:71-80.

16. Heiss C, Jahn S, Taylor M, *et al.* Improvement of endothelial function with dietary flavanols is associated with mobilization of circulating angiogenic cells in patients with coronary artery disease. *J Am Coll Cardiol* 2010;56:218-224.

17. Flammer AJ, Sudano I, Wolfrum M, *et al.* Cardiovascular effects of flavanol-rich chocolate in patients with heart failure. *Eur Heart J* 2011; [epub ahead of print]. doi:10.1093/eurheartj/ehr448.

18. Flammer AJ, Hermann F, Sudano I, *et al.* Dark chocolate improves coronary vasomotion and reduces platelet reactivity. *Circulation* 2007;116: 2376–2382.

19. Loffredo L, Carnevale R, Perri L, *et al.* NOX2-mediated arterial dysfunction in smokers: acute effect of dark chocolate. *Heart* 2011;97:1776-1781.

20. Heiss C, Finis D, Kleinbongard P, *et al.* Sustained increase in flow-mediated dilation after daily intake of high-flavanol cocoa drink over 1 week. *J Cardiovasc Pharmacol* 2007;49:74-80.

21. Heiss C, Kleinbongard P, Dejam A, *et al.* Acute consumption of flavanol-rich cocoa and the reversal of endothelial dysfunction in smokers. *J Am Coll Cardiol* 2005;46:1276-1283.

22. Hermann F, Spieker IE, Ruschitzka F, *et al.* Dark chocolate improves endothelial and platelet function *Heart* 2006;92:119-120.

23. Esser D, Mars M, Oosterink E, *et al.* Dark chocolate consumption improves leukocyte adhesion factors and vascular function in overweight men. *FASEB J.* December 4, 2013; [epub ahead of print]. doi: 10.1096/fj.13-239384.

24. West SG, McIntyre MD, Piotrowski MJ, *et al.* Effects of dark chocolate and cocoa consumption on endothelial function and arterial stiffness in overweight adults. *Br J Nutr* 2014;111:653-661.

25. Faridi Z, Njike VY, Dutta S, *et al.* Acute dark chocolate and cocoa ingestion and endothelial function: a randomized controlled crossover trial *Am J Clin Nutr* 2008;88: 58-63.

CHAPTER 7 REFERENCES

1. Shrime MG, Bauer SR, McDonald AC, *et al.* Flavonoid-rich cocoa consumption affects multiple cardiovascular risk factors in a meta-analysis of short-term studies. *J Nutr* 2011;141:1982-1988.

2. Hooper L, Kay C, Abdelhamid A, *et al.* Effects of chocolate, cocoa, and flavan-3-ols on cardiovascular health: a systematic review and meta-analysis of randomized trials. *Am J Clin Nutr* 2012;95:740-51.

3. Arranz S, Valderas-Martinez P, Chiva-Blanch G, *et al.* Cardioprotective effects of cocoa: Clinical evidence from randomized clinical intervention trials in humans. *Mol Nutr Food Res* 2013;57:936-947.

4. Kwok CS, Boekholdt SM, Lentjes MAH, *et al.* Habitual chocolate consumption and risk of cardiovascular disease among healthy men and women. *Heart* 2014;doi:10.1136/heartjnl-2014-307050.

1. Buitrago-Lopez A, Sanderson J, Johnson L, *et al.* Chocolate consumption and cardiometabolic disorders: systematic review and meta-analysis. *BMJ* 2011;343:d4488doi:10.1136/bmj.d4488.

2. Grassi D, Lippi C, Necozione S, *et al.* Short-term administration of dark chocolate is followed by a significant increase in insulin sensitivity and a decrease in blood pressure in healthy persons. *Am J Clin Nutr* 2005;81:611-614.

3. Hooper L, Kay C, Abdelhamid A, *et al.* Effects of chocolate, cocoa, and flavan-3-ols on cardiovascular health: a systematic review and meta-analysis of randomized trials. *Am J Clin Nutr* 2012;95:740-51.

4. Shrime MG, Bauer SR, McDonald AC, *et al.* Flavonoid-rich cocoa consumption affects multiple cardiovascular risk factors in a meta-analysis of short-term studies. *J Nutr* 2011;141:1982-1988.

5. Lin X, Zhang I, Li A, *et al.* Cocoa flavanol intake and biomarkers for cardiometabolic health: a systematic review and meta-analysis of randomized controlled trials. *J Nutr* 2016;146(11):2325-2333

6. Desideri G, Kwik-Uribe C, Grassi D, *et al.* Benefits in cognitive function, blood pressure and insulin resistance through cocoa flavanol consumption in elderly subjects with mild cognitive impairment: The Cocoa, Cognition, and Aging (CoCoA) study. *Hypertension* 2012;60:794-801.

7. Mastroiacovo D, Kwik-Uribe C, Grassi D, *et al.* Cocoa flavanol consumption improves cognitive function, blood pressure control, and metabolic profile in elderly subjects: Cocoa, Cognition, and Aging (CoCoA) Study–a randomized controlled trial. *Am J Clin Nutr* 2015;101:538-548.

8. Mellor DD, Sathyapalan T, Kilpatrick ES, *et al.* High-cocoa polyphenol-rich chocolate improves HDL cholesterol in Type 2 diabetes patients. *Diabet Med* 2010;27:1318–21.

9. Parsaeyan N, Mozaffari-Khosravi H, Absalan A, *et al.* Beneficial effects of cocoa on lipid peroxidation and inflammatory markers in type 2 diabetic patients and investigation of probable interactions of cocoa active ingredients with prostaglandin synthase-2 (PTGS-2/COX-2) using virtual analysis. *J Diabetes Metab Disord* 2014;13:30.

10. Balzer J, Rassaf T, Heiss C, *et al.* Sustained benefits in vascular function through flavanol-containing cocoa in medicated diabetic patients: a double-masked, randomized, controlled trial. *J Am Coll Cardiol* 2008;51:2141-2149.

11. Mellor DD, Madden LA, Smith KA, *et al.* High-polyphenol chocolate reduces endothelial dysfunction and oxidative stress during acute transient hyperglycaemia in type 2 diabetes: A pilot randomized controlled trial. *Diabet Med* 2013;30:478-83.

12. Grassi D, Necozione S, Lippi C, *et al.* Cocoa reduces blood pressure and insulin resistance and improves endothelium- dependent vasodilation in hypertensives *Hypertension* 2005;46:398-405.

13. Grassi D, Lippi C, Necozione S, *et al.* Short-term administration of dark chocolate is followed by a significant increase in insulin sensitivity and a decrease in blood pressure in healthy persons. *American Society for Clinical Nutrition* 2005;81:611-614.

14. Rostami A, Khalili M, Haghighat N, *et al.* High-cocoa polyphenol-rich chocolate improves blood pressure in patients with diabetes and hypertension. *ARYA Atheroscler* 2015;11(1):21-29

15. Hooper L, Kay C, Abdelhamid A, *et al.* Effects of chocolate, cocoa, and flavan-3-ols on cardiovascular health: a systematic review and meta-analysis of randomized trials. *Am J Clin Nutr* 2012;95:740-51.

16. Zomer E, Owen A, Magliano DJ, *et al.* The effectiveness and cost effectiveness of dark chocolate consumption as prevention therapy in people at high risk of cardiovascular disease: best case scenario analysis using a Markov model. *BMJ* 2012;344:e3657.

17. Grassi D, Desideri G, Necozione S, *et al.* Blood pressure is reduced and insulin sensitivity increased in glucose-intolerant, hypertensive subjects after 15 days of consuming high-polyphenol dark chocolate. *J Nutr* 2008;138:1671-6.

18. Almoosawi S, Fyfe L, Ho C, *et al.* The effect of polyphenol-rich dark chocolate on fasting capillary whole blood glucose, total cholesterol, blood pressure and glucocorticoids in healthy overweight and obese subjects. *Br J Nutr* 2010;103:842-850.

19. Li G, Zhang P, Wang J, *et al.* The long-term effect of lifestyle interventions to prevent diabetes in the China Da Qing Diabetes Prevention Study: a 20-year follow-up study. *Lancet* 2008;371:1783-9.

20. Chandalia M, Garg A, Lutjohann D, *et al.* Beneficial effects of high dietary fibre intake in patients with type 2 diabetes mellitus. *New Engl J Med* 2000;342:1392-98.

21. Anderson JW, Allgood LD, Turner J, *et al.* Effects of psyllium on glucose and serum lipid responses in men with type 2 diabetes and hypercholesterolemia. *Am J Clin Nutr* 1999;70:466-73.

22. Rodríguez-Morán M, Guerrero-Romero F, Lazcano-Burciaga G. Lipid- and glucose-lowering efficacy of plantago psylliumin type II diabetes. *J Diab Comp* 1998;12:273-78.

23. Seyed AZ, Larijani B, Akhoondzadeh S, *et al.* Psyllium decreased serum glucose and glycosylated hemoglobin significantly in diabetic outpatients. *Journal of Ethnopharmacology* 2005;102:202-7.

24. Sierra M, García JJ, Fernández N, *et al.* Therapeutic effects of psyllium in type 2 diabetic patients. *Eur J Clin Nutr* 2002;56:830-42.

25. Landin K, Holm G, Tengborn L, *et al.* Guar gum improves insulin sensitivity, blood lipids, blood pressure, and fibrinolysis in healthy men. *Am J Clin Nutr* 1992;56:1061-65.

26. Schwartz SE, Levine RA, Weinstock RS, *et al.* Sustained pectin ingestion: effect on gastric emptying and glucose tolerance in non-insulin-dependent diabetic patients. *Am J Clin Nutr* 1988;48:1413-17.

27. Hallfrisch J, Scholfield DJ, Behall KM. Diets containing soluble oat extracts improve glucose and insulin responses of moderately hypercholesterolemic men and women. *Am J Clin Nutr* 1995;61:379-84.

28. Barnard ND, Cohen J, Jenkins DJ. A low-fat vegan diet improves glycemic control and cardiovascular risk factors in a randomized clinical trial in individuals with type 2 diabetes. *Diabetes Care* 2006;29:1777-83.

29. Pan A, Sun Q, Bernstein AM, *et al.* Changes in red meat consumption and subsequent risk of type 2 diabetes mellitus: three cohorts of US men and women. *JAMA Intern Med* 2013;173:1328-35.

30. Williams DE, Wareham NJ, Cox BD, *et al.* Frequent salad vegetable consumption is associated with a reduction in the risk of diabetes mellitus. *J Clin Epidemiol* 1999;52:329-35.

31. Cooper AJ, Sharp SJ, Lentjes MA, *et al.* A prospective study of the association between quantity and variety of fruit and vegetable intake and incident type 2 diabetes. *Diabetes Care* 2012;35:1293-300.

32. Nettleton JA, Steffen LM, Ni H, *et al.* Dietary patterns and risk of incident type 2 diabetes I the Multi-Ethnic Study of Atherosclerosis (MESA). *Diabetes Care* 2008;31:1777-82.

33. Pan A, Sun Q, Manson JE, *et al.* Walnut consumption is associated with lower risk of type 2 diabetes in women. *J Nutr* 2013;143:512-8.

34. Wedick NM, Pan A, Cassidy A, *et al.* Dietary flavonoid intakes and risk of type 2 diabetes in US men and women. *Am J Clin Nutr* 2012;95:925-33.

35. Liu YJ, Zhan J, Liu XL, *et al.* Dietary flavonoids intake and risk of type 2 diabetes: a meta-analysis of prospective cohort studies. *Clin Nutr* 2014;33:59-63.

36. Liu K, Zhou R, Wang B, *et al.* Effect of green tea on glucose control and insulin sensitivity: a meta-analysis of 17 randomized controlled trials. *Am J Clin Nutr* 2013;98:340-8.

37. Anderson RA, Polansky MM, Bryden NA, *et al.* Supplemental- chromium effects on glucose, insulin, glucagons, and urinary chromium losses in subjects consuming controlled low-chromium diets. *Am J Clin Nutr* 1991;54:909-16.

38. Mertz W. Chromium in human nutrition: a review. *J Nutr* 1993;123:626-33.

39. Anderson RA, Cheng N, Bryden NA, *et al.* Elevated intakes of supplemental chromium improve glucose and insulin variables in individuals with type 2 diabetes. *Diabetes* 1997;46:1786-91.

40. Fox GN, Sabovic Z. Chromium picolinate supplementation for diabetes mellitus. *J Fam Pract* 1998;46:83-86.

41. Martin J, Wang ZQ, Zhang XH, *et al.* Chromium Picolinate Supplementation Attenuates Body Weight Gain and Increases Insulin Sensitivity in Subjects With Type 2 Diabetes. *Diabetes Care* 2006;29:1826-32.

42. Albarracin CA, Fuqua BC, Evans JL, *et al.* Chromium picolinate and biotin combination improves glucose metabolism in treated uncontrolled overweight to obese patients with type 2 diabetes. *Diabetes Metab Res Rev* 2008;24:41-51.

43. Mooradian AD, Morley JE. Micronutrient status in diabetes mellitus. *Am J Clin Nutr* 1987;45:877-95.

44. Rao KVR, Seshiah V, Kumar TV. Effect of zinc sulfate therapy on control and lipids in type I diabetes. *J Assoc Physicians India* 1987;35:52.

45. Harding AH, Wareham NJ, Bingham SA, *et al.* Plasma vitamin C level, fruit and vegetable consumption, and the risk of new-onset type 2 diabetes mellitus: the European prospective investigation of cancer—Norfolk prospective study. *Arch Intern Med* 2008;168:1493-9.

46. Adv Pharm Sci 2011; doi:10.1155/2011/195271.

47. Mooren FC, Krüger K, Völker K, *et al.* Oral magnesium supplementation reduces insulin resistance in non-diabetic subjects—a double-blind, placebo-controlled, randomized trial. *Diabetes Obes Metab* 2011;13:281-4.

48. Sjorgren A, Floren CH, Nilsson A. Oral administration of magnesium hydroxide to subjects with insulin dependent diabetes mellitus. *Magnesium* 1988;121:16-20.

49. Paolisso G, Sgambato S, Pizza G, *et al.* Improved insulin response and action by chronic magnesium administration in aged NIDDM subjects. *Diabetes Care* 1989;12:265-69.

50. Chiu KC. Hypovitaminosis D is associated with insulin resistance and beta cell dysfunction. *Am J Clin Nutr* 2004;79:820-25.

51. Hyppönen E, Läärä E, Reunanen A, *et al.* Intake of vitamin D and risk of type 1 diabetes: a birth-cohort study. *Lancet* 2001;358:1500-03.

52. Littorin B, Blom P, Schölin A *et al.* Lower levels of plasma 25-hydroxyvitamin D among young adults at diagnosis of autoimmune type 1 diabetes compared with control subjects: results from the nationwide Diabetes Incidence Study in Sweden (DISS). *Diabetologia* 2006; 49:2847-52.

53. Hyppönen E, Läärä E, Reunanen A, *et al.* Intake of vitamin D and risk of type 1 diabetes: a birth-cohort study. *Lancet* 2001;358:1500-03.

54. McCarty MF. Can correction of sub-optimal coenzyme Q status improve beta-cell function in type II diabetics? *Med Hypotheses* 1999;52:397-400.

55. Jacob S, Ruus P, Hermann R, *et al.* Oral administration of RAC-alpha-lipoic acid modulates insulin sensitivity in patients with type-2 diabetes mellitus: a placebo-controlled pilot trial. *Free Radic Biol Med* 1999;27:309-14.

56. Khan A, Safdar M, Khan MMA, *et al.* Cinnamon improves glucose and lipids of people with type 2 diabetes. *Diabetes Care* 2003;26:3215-8.

57. Lua T, Shenga H, Johnna W, *et al.* Cinnamon Extract Improves Fasting Blood Glucose and Glycosylated Hemoglobin Level in Chinese Patients with Type 2 Diabetes. *Nutr Res* 2012;32:408-12.

58. Hlebowicz J, Darwiche G, Björgell O, *et al.* Effect of cinnamon on postprandial blood glucose, gastric emptying, and satiety in healthy subjects. *Am J Clin Nutr* 2007;85:1552-6.

59. Mang B, Wolters M, Schmitt B, *et al.* Effects of a cinnamon extract on plasma glucose, HbA, and serum lipids in diabetes mellitus type 2. *Eur J Clin Invest* 2006;36:340-4.

60. Davis PA, Yokoyama W. Cinnamon intake lowers fasting blood glucose: meta-analysis. *J Med Food* 2011;14:884-9.

61. Allen RW, Schwartzmann E, Baker WL, *et al.* Cinnamon use in type 2 Diabetes: an updated systematic review and meta-analysis. *Ann Fam Med* 2013;11:452-9.

62. Sharma RD, Raghuram TC, Rao NS. Effect of fenugreek seeds on blood glucose and serum lipids in type 1 diabeties. *Eur J Clin Nutr* 1990;44:301-6.

63. Madar Z, Abel R, Samish S, *et al.* Glucose-lowering effect of fenugreek in non-insulin dependent diabetics. *Eur J Clin Nutr* 1988;42:51-4.

64. Sharma RD, Sakar A, Hazra DK, *et al.* Use of fenugreek seed powder in the management of non-insulin dependent diabetes mellitus. *Nutr Res* 1996;16:1131-9.

65. Lu FR, Shen L, Qin Y, *et al.* Clinical observation on trigonella foenum-graecum L. total saponins in combination with sulfonylureas in the treatment of type 2 diabetes mellitus. *Chin J Integr Med* 2008;14:56-60.

66. Ashraf R, Khan RA, Ashraf I. Garlic (Allium sativum) supplementation with standard antidiabetic agent provides better diabetic control in type 2 diabetes patients. *Pak J Pharm Sci* 2011;24:565-70.

67. Shidfar F, Rajab A,Rahideh T, *et al.* The effect of ginger (Zingiber officinale) on glycemic markers in patients with type 2 diabetes. *J Compliment Integr Med* 2015;12:165-70.

68. Welihinda J, Karunanayake EH, Sheriff MH, *et al.* Effect of Momordica charantia on the glucose tolerance in maturity onset diabetes. *J Ethnopharmacol* 1986;17:277-82.

69. Srivastava Y, Venkatakrishna-Bhatt H, Verma Y, *et al.* Anti-diabetic and adaptogenic properties of Momordica charantia extract: an experimental and clinical evaluation. *Phytother Res* 1993;7:285–9.

70. Shanmugasundaram ER, Rajeswari G, Baskaran K, *et al.* Use of Gymnema sylvestre leaf extract in the control of blood glucose in insulin-dependent diabetes mellitus. *J Ethnopharmacol* 1990;30:281-94.

71. Baskaran K, Kizar Ahamath B, Radha Shanmugasundaram K, *et al.* Antidiabetic effect of a leaf extract from *Gymnema sylvestre* in non-insulin-dependent diabetes mellitus patients. *J Ethnopharmacol* 1990;30:295-30.

72. Yin J, Xing H, Ye J. Efficacy of berberine in patients with type 2 diabetes mellitus. *Metabolism* 2008;57:712-17.

73. Zhang H, Wei J, Xue R, *et al.* Berberine lowers blood glucose in type 2 diabetes mellitus patients through increasing insulin receptor expression. *Metabolism* 2010;59:285-92.

74. Li D, Zhang Y, Liu Y, *et al.* Purified Anthocyanin Supplementation Reduces Dyslipidemia, Enhances Antioxidant Capacity, and Prevents Insulin Resistance in Diabetic Patients. *J Nutr* 2015.doi:10.3945/jn.114.205674.

1. Nurk E, Refsum H, Drevon CA, *et al.* Intake of flavonoid-rich wine, tea, and chocolate by elderly men and women is associated with better cognitive test performance. *J Nutr* 2009;139:120-7.

2. Moreira A, Diógenes MJ, de Mendonça A, *et al.* Chocolate Consumption is Associated with a Lower Risk of Cognitive Decline. *J Alzheimers Dis* 2016;53(1):85-93.

3. Sorond FA, Lipsitz LA, Hollenberg NK, *et al.* Cerebral blood flow response to flavanol-rich cocoa in healthy elderly humans. *Neuropsychiatr Dis Treat* 2008;4:433-440.

4. Brickman AM, Khan UA, Provenzano FA, *et al.* Enhancing dentate gyrus function with dietary flavanols improves cognition in older adults. *Nature Neuroscience* 2014;17:1798-1803.

5. Field DT, Williams CM, Butler LT. Consumption of cocoa flavanols results in an acute improvement in visual and cognitive functions. *Physiol Behav* 2011;103):255-260.

6. Mastroiacovo D, Kwik-Uribe C, Grassi D, *et a*l. Cocoa flavanol consumption improves cognitive function, blood pressure control, and metabolic profile in elderly subjects: the Cocoa, Cognition, and Aging (CoCoA) Study–a randomized controlled trial. *Am J Clin Nutr* 2015;101:538-548.

7. Tricco AC, Soobiah C, Berliner S, *et al.* Efficacy and safety of cognitive enhancers for patients with mild cognitive impairment: a systematic review and meta-analysis. *CMAJ* 2013;185:1393-1401.

8. Desideri G, Kwik-Uribe C, Grassi D, *et al.* Benefits in cognitive function, blood pressure and insulin resistance through cocoa flavanol consumption in elderly subjects with mild cognitive impairment: The Cocoa, Cognition, and Aging (CoCoA) study. *Hypertension* 2012;60:794-801.

9. Macht M, Mueller J. Immediate effects of chocolate on experimentally induced mood states. *Appetite* 2007;49:667-74.

10. Pase MP, Scholey AB, Pipingas A, *et al.* Cocoa polyphenols enhance positive mood states but not cognitive performance: A randomized, placebo-controlled trial. *J Psychopharmacol* 2013;27:451-8.

11. Scholey AB, French SJ, Morris PJ, *et al.* Consumption of cocoa flavanols results in acute improvements in mood and cognitive performance during sustained mental effort. *J Psychopharm* 2009;doi:10.1177/0269881109106923.

12. Martin F-PJ, Rezzi S, Peré-Trepat E, *et al.* Metabolic effects of dark chocolate consumption on energy, gut microbiota, and stress-related metabolism in free-living subjects. *J Proteome Res* 2009;8:5568-79.

13. Wirtz PH, von Känel R, Meister RE, *et al.* Dark chocolate intake buffers stress reactivity in humans. *J Am Coll Cardiol* 2014;63:2297-2299.

14. Kuebler U, Arpagaus A, Meister RE, *et al.* Dark chocolate attenuates intracellular pro-inflammatory reactivity to acute psychosocial stress in men: A randomized controlled trial. *Brain Behav Immun* 2016;pii:S0889-1591(16)30097-6.

1. Davison K, Coates AM, Buckley JD, *et al.* Effect of cocoa flavanols and exercise on cardiometabolic risk factors in overweight and obese subjects. *Int J Obes* **(Lond)** 2008;32:1289-1296.

2. Mellor DD, Sathyapalan T, Kilpatrick ES, *et al.* High-cocoa polyphenol-rich chocolate improves HDL cholesterol in Type 2 diabetes patients. *Diabet Med* 2010;27:1318–21.

3. Golomb BA, Koperski S, White HL. Association between more frequent chocolate consumption and lower body mass index. *Arch Intern Med* 2012;172:519-21.

4. Cuenca-Garcia M, Ruiz JR, Ortega FB, *et al.* Association between chocolate consumption and fatness in European adolescents. *Nutrition* 2014;30:236-9.

5. Di Renzo L, Rizzo M, Sarlo C, *et al.* Effects of dark chocolate in a population of Normal Weight Obese women: a pilot study. *Eur Rev Med Pharmacol Sci* 2013;17:2257-66.

6. Bohannon J, Koch D, Homm P, *et al.* Chocolate with high cocoa content as a weight-loss accelerator. *International Archives of Medicine* 2015;8(55).

1. Vertuani S, Scalambra E, Vittorio T, *et al.* Evaluation of antiradical activity of different cocoa and chocolate products: relation with lipid and protein composition. *J Med Food* 2014;17:512-516.

2. Miller KB, Hurst WJ, Flannigan N, *et al.* Survey of commercially available chocolate- and cocoa-containing products in the United States. 2. Comparison of flavan-3-ol content with nonfat cocoa solids, total polyphenols, and percent cacao. J *Agric Food Chem* 2009;57:9169-9180.

3. Scheid L, Reusch A, Stehle P, *et al.* Antioxidant effects of cocoa and cocoa products ex vivo and in vivo: is there evidence from controlled intervention studies? *Curr Opin Clin Nutr Metab Care* 2010;13:737-42.

4. Baba S, Natsume M, Yasuda A, *et al.* Plasma LDL and HDL cholesterol and oxidized LDL concentrations are altered in normo- and hypercholesterolemic humans after intake of different levels of cocoa powder. *J Nutr* 2007;137:1436-41.

5. Nanetti L, Vignini A, Gregori A, *et al.* Effect of consumption of dark chocolate on lipoproteins and serum lipids. *Mederranean Journal of Nutrition and Metabolism* 2008;1:25-31.

6. Nanetti L, Raffaelli F, Tranquilli AL, **et al**. Effect of consumption of dark chocolate on oxidative stress in lipoproteins and platelets in women and in men. **Appetite** 2012;58:400-405.

7. Arranz S, Valderas-Martinez P, Chiva-Blanch G, *et al.* Cardioprotective effects of cocoa: Clinical evidence from randomized clinical intervention trials in humans. *Mol Nutr Food Res* 2013;57:936-947.

8. Spadafranca A, Martinez Conesa C, Sirini S, *et al.* Effect of dark chocolate on plasma epicatechin levels, DNA resistance to oxidative stress and total antioxidant activity in healthy subjects. *Br J Nutr* 2010;103:1008-1014.

9. Engler M, Engler M, Chen C, *et al.* Flavonoid-rich dark chocolate improves endothelial function and increases plasma epicatechin concetrations in healthy adults *J Am Coll Nutr* 2004;23:197-204.

10. Wan Y, Vinson JA, Etherton TD, *et al.* Effects of cocoa powder and dark chocolate on LDL oxidative susceptibility and prostaglandin concentrations in humans. *Am J Clin Nutr* 2001;74:596-602.

11. Allgrove J, Farrell E, Gleeson M, *et al.* Regular dark chocolate consumption's reduction of oxidative stress and increase of free-fatty-acid mobilization in response to prolonged cycling. *Int J Sport Nutr Exerc Metab* 2011;21:113-23.

12. Hermann F, Spieker IE, Ruschitzka F, *et al.* Dark chocolate improves endothelial and platelet function *Heart* 2006;92:119-120.

13. Loffredo L, Del Ben M, Perri L, *et al.* Effects of dark chocolate on NOX-2-generated oxidative stress in patients with non-alcoholic steatohepatitis. *Aliment Pharmacol Ther* 2016;44(3):279-286.

14. Thomas K, Morris P, Stevenson E. Improved endurance capacity following chocolate milk consumption compared with 2 commercially available sport drinks. *Applied Physiology, Nutrition, and Metabolism* 2009;34:78-82.

15. Patel RK, Brouner J, Spendiff O. Dark chocolate supplementation reduces the oxygen cost of moderate intensity cycling. *J Int Soc Sports Nutr* 2015;15;12:47.

16. Tsukamoto H, Suga T, Ishibashi A, *et al.* Flavanol-rich cocoa consumption enhances exercise-induced executive function improvements in humans. *Nutrition* 2018;46:90-6.

17. di Giuseppe R, Di Castelnuovo A, Centritto F, *et al.* Regular consumption of dark chocolate is associated with low serum concentrations of C-reactive protein in a healthy Italian population. *J Nutr* 2008;138:1939-1945.

18. Monagas A, Khan N, Andres-Lacueva C, *et al.* Effect of cocoa powder on the modulation of inflammatory biomarkers in patients at high risk of cardiovascular disease. *Am J Clin Nutr* 2009;90:1144-50.

19. Tzounis X, Rodriguez-Mateos A, Vulevic J, *et al.*. Prebiotic evaluation of cocoa-derived flavanols in healthy humans by using a randomized, controlled, double-blind, crossover intervention study. *Am J Clin Nutr* 2011;93:62–72.

20. Lin X, Zhang I, Li A, *et al.* Cocoa flavanol intake and biomarkers for cardiometabolic health: a systematic review and meta-analysis of randomized controlled trials. *J Nutr* 2016;146(11):2325-2333.

21. Kuebler U, Arpagaus A, Meisger RE, *et al.* Dark chocolate attenuates intracellular pro-inflammatory reactivity to acute psychosocial stress in men: A randomized controlled trial. *Brain Behav Immun* 2016;pii:S0889-1591(16)30097-6.

22. Triche EW, Grosso LM, Belanger K, *et al.* Chocolate consumption in pregnancy and reduced likelihood of preeclampsia. *Epidemiol* 2008;19:459-64.

23. Saftlas AF, Triche EW, Beydoun H, *et al.* Does chocolate intake during pregnancy reduce the risks of preeclampsia and gestational hypertension? *Ann Epidemiol* 2010;20:584-591.

24. Di Renzo GC, Brillo E, Romanelli M, *et al.* Potential effects of chocolate on human pregnancy: a randomized controlled trial. *J Matern Fetal Neonatal Med.* 2012;25:1860-1867.

25. Tzounis X, Rodriguez-Mateos A, Vulevic J, *et al.*. Prebiotic evaluation of cocoa-derived flavanols in healthy humans by using a randomized, controlled, double-blind, crossover intervention study. *Am J Clin Nutr* 2011;93:62–72.

26. Sarriá B, Martínez-López S, Fernández-Espinosa A, *et al.*. Effects of regularly consuming dietary fibre rich soluble cocoa products on bowel habits in healthy subjects: a free-living, two-stage, randomized, crossover, single-blind intervention. *Nutr Metab* 2012;9:33.

27. Castillejo G, Bullo M, Anguera A, *et al.*. A controlled randomized, double-blind trial to evaluate the effect of a supplement of cocoa husk that is rich in dietary fiber on colonic transit in constipated pediatric patients. *Pediatrics* 2006;118:e641-e648.

28. Sathyapalan T, Beckett S, Rigby AS, *et al.* High cocoa polyphenol rich chocolate may reduce the burden of the symptoms in chronic fatigue syndrome. *Nutr J* 2010;9:55.

29. Heinrich U, Neukan K, Tronnier H, *et al.* Long-term ingestion of high flavanol cocoa provides photoprotection against UV-induced erythema and improves skin condition in women. *J Nutr* 2006;136:1565-9.

30. Williams S, tamburic S, Lally C. Eating chocolate can significantly protect the skin from UV light. *Lett Appl Microbiol* 2009;49:354-60.

31. Yoon H-S, Kim JR, Park GY, *et al.* Cocoa Flavanol Supplementation Influences Skin Conditions of Photo-Aged Women: A 24-Week Double-Blind, Randomized, Controlled Trial. *J Nutr* 2015;doi:10.3945/jn.115.217711.

32. Srikanth RK, Shashikiran ND, Subba Reddy VV. Chocolate mouth rinse: effect on plaque accumulation and mutans streptococci counts when used by children. *J Indian Soc Pedod Prevent Dent* 2008:66-70.

33. Rabin JC, Karunathilake N, Patrizi K. Effects of Milk vs Dark Chocolate Consumption on Visual Acuity and Contrast Sensitivity Within 2 Hours: A Randomized Clinical Trial. *JAMA Opthalmol* 2018;doi:10.1001/jamaophthalmol.2018.0978.

34. Field DT, Williams CM, Butler LT. Consumption of cocoa flavanols results in an acute improvement in visual and cognitive functions. *Physiol Behav* 2011;103:255-260.